Midwives, Research and Childbirth

VOLUME 1

Midwives, Research and Childbirth

VOLUME 1

Edited by

Sarah Robinson

Senior Research Fellow, Nursing Research Unit
King's College, London

and

Ann M. Thomson

Clinical Lecturer, Department of Nursing
University of Manchester
Midwifery Sister, St Mary's Hospital, Manchester

London   New York
CHAPMAN AND HALL

For Anne Bent

First published in 1989 by Chapman and Hall Ltd
11 New Fetter Lane, London EC4P 4EE
Published in the USA by Chapman and Hall
29 West 35th Street, New York NY 10001

© 1989 Sarah Robinson and Ann M. Thomson

Printed in Great Britain by
St. Edmundsbury Press Ltd
Bury St. Edmunds, Suffolk
Typeset in $9^{1}/_{2}/11$ Times Roman by
Leaper and Gard Ltd, Bristol

ISBN   0 412 33370 8

British Library Cataloguing in Publication Data

Midwives, research and childbirth.
Vol. 1
1. Women, Pregnancy & childbirth
I. Title   II. Thomson, Ann M.,   *1944-*
618.2

ISBN   0-412-33370-8

Library of Congress Cataloging in Publication Data

Midwives, research and childbirth.
Bibliography: p.
Includes index.
1. Prenatal care.   2. Childbirth.   3. Midwives.
I. Robinson, Sarah, 1948-   .   II. Thomson, Ann M.,
1944-   .
RG940.M53   1988   618.2   88-22852
ISBN   0-412-33370-8 (pbk.)

Contents

Contents

Preface

This volume is the first in a series which brings together studies of particular relevance to the care provided by midwives for childbearing women and their families. The series is intended primarily for midwives but we hope that other health professionals involved in the maternity services, as well as those who use the services, will also find the series interesting and useful.

In undertaking this venture we have been fortunate in the support received from colleagues, friends and family. In particular we would like to thank the following: the editorial and production staff at Chapman and Hall in London for encouragement and advice; all the authors who have contributed to the series; colleagues at both the Nursing Research Unit, London University and the Department of Nursing Studies, Manchester University; and Paul and Rachel Robinson.

This first volume is dedicated to Anne Bent, formerly Director of Education at the Royal College of Midwives and then Professional Officer for Midwifery at the United Kingdom Central Council for Nursing, Midwifery and Health Visiting. Always conscious of the need for midwifery to become a research-based profession and for midwives to be aware of the importance of research, she has made a major contribution to initiating and facilitating developments in both these respects.

Sarah Robinson, *London*
Ann M. Thomson, *Manchester*
February 1988

Contributors

Jean A. Ball	Lecturer in Quality Assurance, Nuffield Institute for Health Care Services, Leeds University
Sheila Drayton	Head Midwife, Gwent Health Authority
Mavis Kirkham	Midwifery Sister, Netheredge Hospital, Sheffield
Maureen Laryea	Lecturer, Institute of Nursing Studies, University of Hull
Sally Macintyre	Director, Medical Research Council, Medical Sociology Unit, Glasgow
James McIntosh	Lecturer, Department of Social Administration, University of Glasgow
Rosemary Methven	Senior Midwifery Tutor, Post-Basic Studies, Clarendon Wing of Leeds Royal Infirmary
Maureen Porter	Honorary Research Fellow, Department of Sociology, University of Aberdeen
Jean Proud	Senior Midwife Ultrasonographer, Peterborough Maternity Unit
Colin Rees	Lecturer in Research and Sociology, South Glamorgan School of Nursing
Sarah Robinson	Senior Research Fellow, Nursing Research Unit, King's College, University of London
Ann M. Thomson	Clinical Lecturer, Department of Nursing, University of Manchester/Midwifery Sister, St Mary's Hospital, Manchester

CHAPTER ONE

Research and midwifery

Sarah Robinson and Ann M. Thomson

THE SCOPE OF MIDWIFERY RESEARCH

This series starts from the premise that midwives in Britain are qualified to provide care on their own responsibility throughout pregnancy, labour and the puerperium, to recognize those signs of abnormality that require referral to medical staff, and to provide advice, information and support from early pregnancy to the end of the postnatal period. The brief for a series focusing on midwifery is therefore necessarily wide, as midwifery is concerned with all the main elements of maternity care, the clinical, the advisory and the supportive. Many of the studies included in the series focus on specific aspects of this care; they include the evaluation of long-standing practices as well as more recently introduced innovations.

As a profession, midwifery has experienced many constraints on the opportunities available for its members to fulfil the role for which they are qualified. In particular, increasing medical involvement in normal maternity care and the fragmentation of this care between a number of health professionals have led to much concern and dissatisfaction (Royal College of Midwives, 1977; Cowell and Wainwright, 1981; Robinson *et al.*, 1983; Towler and Brammall, 1986). Some of the studies in this series focus on the effects of these constraints on the role of the midwife. Others seek to evaluate whether care provided primarily by medical staff compared with care provided primarily by midwives has any advantages in terms of perinatal and neonatal outcomes and satisfaction with the experience of childbirth.

The series focuses on midwives themselves as well as on midwifery practice. If midwives are to make their full contribution to the care of women during pregnancy and childbirth, a high standard of educational preparation is required as are a career structure and conditions of service that encourage recruitment to and retention in the profession. Several studies that focus on aspects of midwifery education and on career patterns of midwives have been undertaken or are in progress, and will be included in volumes 2 and 3 of the series.

Women's views and experiences of maternity care have been the subject of much research in recent years and the findings of these studies often have important implications for midwifery practice. They identify sources of consumer satisfaction and dissatisfaction with the service and also indicate ways in which midwifery skills and knowledge can be more appropriately deployed in meeting women's needs. The series therefore includes studies that have focused specifically on women's views and experiences of maternity care as well as those that have included women's views as part of wider investigations.

OPPORTUNITIES FOR MIDWIFERY RESEARCH

During the 1970s, the view steadily gained ground that midwifery practice and education should be based on research findings rather than on custom and tradition or the dictates of other professional groups. Prior to this time, a number of projects had been undertaken but were few and far between. One of the earliest was a survey of midwives' reasons for taking training and their responsibilities once in post (Ministry of Health *et al.*, 1949). Undertaken as part of an investigation into the shortage of midwives prevailing in the 1940s, this study highlighted the extent to which the role of the midwife, with its focus on the normality of child-birth, was being overshadowed by an increasing focus on potential ab-normalities. A later study (Ramsden and Radwanski, 1963) showed that, as in the 1940s, many midwives obtained a midwifery qualification to enhance their nursing career prospects and not because they wished to practise midwifery. The interrelationship between the responsibilities of midwives and medical staff was explored in a small scale study by Walker in 1972 (Walker, 1976) and the mid-1970s saw the publication of several studies that sought to determine the number of midwives required to staff the maternity services (Sheffield Regional Hospital Board, 1972; Auld, 1974; Croydon Area Health Authority, 1976; Papakyriakou, 1977).

From the mid-1970s onwards, a growing number of studies were undertaken, focusing primarily on midwifery practice, but also on aspects of education and management as well. This was a reflection of the increasing opportunities available to midwives, and other professionals, who wished to pursue research in this area. These opportunities included Department of Health and Social Security (DHSS) and Scottish Home and Health Department (SHHD) research studentships and scholarships awarded by companies such as Maws. In addition, an increasing number of midwives researched aspects of midwifery for their undergraduate and post-graduate dissertations. Research undertaken by these means tended to be single projects. However, longer-term programmes of research into aspects of midwifery were also established in the late 1970s, mainly located in DHSS-funded units such as the Nursing Research Unit at King's College (formerly Chelsea College), London University and the National Perinatal Epidemiology Unit in Oxford. Staff at some hospitals also developed a programme of practice research; the best-known example in this respect is probably the team at Northwick Park Hospital where midwives and obstetricians have collaborated on a series of studies.

Research undertaken in all these situations (degrees, scholarships and unit programmes) are included in this series of books.

SUPPORT FOR AND DISSEMINATION OF MIDWIFERY RESEARCH

If a profession is to develop a research base successfully, it requires not only practitioners willing to undertake research but also colleagues who are willing to support them in the process and a programme of dissemination and implementation of findings. As Brotherston (1964) has argued, this in turn requires a 'research awareness' in the body of the profession who may not be undertaking research themselves. Midwifery has sought to increase this 'research awareness' through research appreciation refresher courses, research methods courses for tutors and an increasing research component in basic and post-basic midwifery education. Individual midwives have had opportunities to attain skills by means of post-basic and post-graduate research methods courses and through the experience of holding scholarships or joining research teams.

Evidence of a commitment to dissemination of research findings is now demonstrated by a number of developments: these include the annual 'Research and the Midwife' conferences; the Royal College of Midwives Current Awareness Bulletin; the Midwives' Information and Resource Service (MIDIRS); and the publication of new journals. The availability of publications on research relevant to midwifery has, to some extent, been problematic. Some projects are only available as reports with a limited circulation, or as short papers in conference proceedings. Others are included in collections of readings on topics as diverse as nursing, and the sociology of childbirth. We think there is a need for a series of books which brings these studies together and into a format which provides authors with the opportunity to describe their methods and findings in some detail.

In selecting studies for the series, our policy is for each volume to include studies which together encompass a wide range of aspects of midwifery – policies and practices, inter and intra professional relationships, education and management. In this first volume we have included some of the earlier studies undertaken. This is for two reasons: first, to make them more widely available than hitherto; secondly, so that in due course the series will constitute a comprehensive record of research in this area, with earlier studies available as bench marks against which later work may be compared.

Inevitably, editors in any field have guidelines that help to provide consistency throughout a volume. As this volume is based on the premise that midwives are qualified to provide care for normal childbearing women, we have presumed these women not to be sick and have therefore not labelled them as 'patients'. We have included the term 'patients' when this is how the women were seen to be treated by those providing their care, but we have put it in parentheses as, for example, in Kirkham's and Drayton and Rees' chapters. We have followed the tradition that uses the term 'obstetrics' as applied to care in childbirth provided by doctors, and 'midwifery' as applied to care in childbirth provided by midwives. The terms 'monitor' and 'monitoring' have been used to indicate the midwife's use of all her senses and skills in assessing the progress of the woman and the fetus/baby throughout pregnancy, labour and the puerperium. It should not be interpreted as referring only to the use of continual fetal heart rate monitoring machines. The terms 'booking interview' and 'booking' are used in several of the chapters; this is a shorthand phrase used in midwifery and obstetrics, and refers to the woman's first visit to the antenatal clinic to book (i.e. reserve) a bed.

RESEARCH STRATEGIES

Midwifery is often described as an art and a science: as such, a diversity of research strategies and methods are appropriate for its study. These range from randomized controlled trials to evaluate the effects of clinical procedures to detailed observational studies to describe interactions between midwives and the women in their care; the studies included in the first volume illustrate this diversity. Each of the authors has described his or her research design, the process of negotiating access to carry out the study and the methods of analysis in some detail, in order to indicate routes that others may follow and difficulties they may encounter.

The study by Robinson (Chapter 1) involved a national survey by questionnaire of several thousand health professionals. This was in order to obtain data from a wide range of settings about a subject on which little prior information existed, namely the level of responsibility exercised by midwives. Two studies, those by Proud (Chapter 5) and by Drayton and Rees (Chapter 7), took the form of randomized controlled trials. The first investigated whether clinical actions taken on the basis of placental grading improved perinatal outcomes; the second investigated the effect of enemas given in labour. Both describe difficulties involved in mounting trials of this kind and in ensuring that trial protocol and consistency in clinical actions are adhered to throughout the course of the study.

Semi-structured or structured interviews as a means of obtaining data on views and experiences of midwives and/or women were used in several of the studies, both prospective and retrospective, in this volume. These include Methven's study of the antenatal booking interview (Chapter 3), Drayton and Rees' study of women's views of enemas (Chapter 7), McIntosh's study of women's expectations and experiences of childbirth (Chapter 10) and Thomson's study of women's intentions in respect of baby feeding (Chapter 11).

Observation was chosen as the main method of investigation by Kirkham in her study of interaction during labour and delivery (Chapter 6), by Porter and Macintyre in their studies of interactions in antenatal clinics and postnatal wards and clinics (Chapter 4) and by Laryea (Chapter 9) in her study of events on postnatal wards. Some studies have employed only one method, others a combination. Ball, for example, used a combination of observation, questionnaire, interviews and medical records in her study of adjustment to motherhood (Chapter 8) and Methven a combination of observation, interviews and questionnaires in her study of information obtained in the course of the antenatal booking interview (Chapter 3).

COMMON THEMES AND ISSUES

Although each of the chapters is complete in itself, several common themes and issues arise from the volume.

Communication

Communication between women and their care-givers is the main focus of several of the chapters. All the studies that involved asking women for their views and experiences of pregnancy and childbirth demonstrate that the availability of information is a central concern. The studies by Methven (Chapter 3) and by Porter and Macintyre (Chapter 4) show that during pregnancy women seek information about health care, about preparation for feeding, and about the place and nature of their delivery. Kirkham (Chapter 6) and McIntosh (Chapter 10) both show that during labour women want to be kept informed of their progress and be told why certain procedures are being carried out. Similarly, Ball (Chapter 8), Laryea (Chapter 9) and Thomson (Chapter 11) show that in the post-natal period, women want consistent advice about feeding and health care. A particular point of interest in this respect emerges from the studies by Kirkham and McIntosh. Some of the midwives studied by Kirkham seemed to hold the view that working-class women did not need or understand information as much as their middle-class counterparts, yet McIntosh's study of working-class primiparae demonstrated a great desire on the part of these women to be kept fully informed of their progress in labour.

Data from the studies that focused on communication led the authors to conclude that many midwives and doctors have poor interviewing techniques, based on a closed style of questioning. This style did not encourage women to articulate their concerns and tended to be dismissive of them when they did. Both Methven, and Porter and Macintyre found that women sometimes appeared to be satisfied with a quality of inter-viewing and information-giving which the researchers, on the basis of observation of the encounter, judged to be poor. As Porter and Macintyre (1984) have suggested, women may be satisfied with what is on offer in the absence of an alternative. A similar point is developed in Drayton and Rees' study, women accept procedures such as enemas because they have been subjected to them in the past and take the view that 'the professionals know what is best'.

Individualization of care

'Routine' is an adjective that has been used to describe many aspects of care provided by midwives in the past and unfortunately is still used today. Chambers' *Dictionary* defines routine as 'regular, unvarying or mechanical course of action or round'. The use of the nursing process has demonstrated how individuals vary and how care needs to be tailored to an individual's needs. The chapters by Methven, Kirkham, Ball and McIntosh highlight the potential value to childbearing women of care that is based on their particular needs and wishes rather than on a 'mechanical course of action'.

Constraints

As noted at the beginning of this chapter, the midwife's role has been subject to a number of constraints and the extent to which medical staff have become involved in normal maternity care has been of particular concern. The chapter by Robinson (Chapter 2) describes a survey of the profession undertaken in 1979 when this concern was at its height. The study documents the ways in which the midwife's level of decision-making had been reduced, particularly in the antenatal period. It also demonstrated that midwifery and medical staff often held differing perceptions of their respective responsibilities for maternity care, and that many midwives appeared to be satisfied with a level of responsibility well below the one for which they are qualified. Later studies, which examine whether these constraints have changed or not, will be included in subsequent volumes.

As some of the respondents in Robinson's study indicated, these constraints lead to a loss of confidence and a subsequent unwillingness to take responsibility. This point was highlighted in the studies by Methven and by Porter and Macintyre, with midwives handing decisions over to medical staff which they might well have been able to make themselves. Similarly, Kirkham concludes that one of the reasons why midwives may be poor at giving information to women in labour is that they themselves are unhappy with policies they are required to implement concerning the management of labour.

Innovations and opportunities

The recent history of midwifery, however, has seen many innovations in care as well as constraints. Methven's work, for example, shows how the use of a nursing process approach to the antenatal booking interview can enable the midwife to obtain a wealth of information relevant to a woman's subsequent care, which fails to emerge in the course of the standard, obstetrically-oriented interview. Later volumes in particular will include studies of innovations in midwifery that have been introduced in recent years.

Many of the studies in the present volume point to areas in which an increase in midwifery knowledge and skills is needed, for example, in interviewing and information-giving. Others provide an indication of how existing knowledge and skills can be used more effectively, for example, in identifying women at risk of emotional distress postpartum and in building up women's confidence in their ability to feed and care for their new baby. In looking to the future, an ongoing programme of evaluation of practice and education needs to be maintained if midwives are to provide childbearing women and their families with effective and satisfying care.

REFERENCES

Auld, M. (1974) *How many nurses?* Royal College of Nursing, London.

Brotherston, J. (1964) *Research-mindedness and the health professionals.* Report of international seminar on research in nursing held by the International Council of Nurses, Geneva.

Cowell, B. and Wainwright, D. (1981) *Behind the Blue Door: The History of the Royal College of Midwives 1881–1981.* Bailliere Tindall, London.

Croydon Area Health Authority (1976) *The use of the qualified midwife.* Croydon Area Health Authority.

Ministry of Health, Department of Health for Scotland, Ministry of Labour and National Service (1949) *Report of the Working Party on Midwives.* HMSO, London.

Papakyriakou, J.K. (1977) A qualitative examination of some of the factors relevant to the determination of a Manpower Planning Policy for Midwives at a health district level. MSc. thesis, Department of Management Studies, University of Manchester Institute for Science and Technology.

Porter, M. and Macintyre, S. (1984) 'What is, must be best': A research note on conservative or deferential responses to antenatal care provision. *Social Science and Medicine, 19* (11), 1197–1200.

Ramsden, P. and Radwanski, P. (1963) *Some aspects of the work of the midwife.* The Dan Mason Nursing Research Committee of the National Florence Nightingale Committee, London.

Robinson, S., Golden, J. and Bradley, S. (1983) *A study of the role and responsibilities of the midwife.* NERU Report no. 1, Chelsea College, London University.

Royal College of Midwives (1977) *Evidence to the Royal Commission on the National Health Service.* Royal College of Midwives, London.

Sheffield Regional Hospital Board (1972) *Report of the Working Party to Study the Hospital Midwife.* Sheffield R.H.B.

Towler, J. and Brammall, J. (1986) *The midwife in history and society.* Croom Helm, Kent.

Walker, J.F. (1976) Midwife or obstetric nurse? Some perceptions of midwives and obstetricians of the role of the midwife. *Journal of Advanced Nursing, 1,* (2), 129–38.

CHAPTER TWO

Caring for childbearing women: the interrelationship between midwifery and medical responsibilities

Sarah Robinson

The role that midwives should fulfil in the maternity services has been the subject of much debate in the last decade, particularly in Europe and North America. This debate has had two main foci. First, differing views concerning the nature of childbirth have led to considerable disagreement about the appropriate roles to be fulfilled by the various professionals involved in maternity care. On the one hand, there has been an emphasis on childbirth as an essentially natural process to be assisted by midwives in their capacity as providers of normal maternity care, albeit with access to obstetric specialists as and when necessary. In contrast, others have focused on the potential abnormalities of childbirth, regarding it as a process requiring ongoing specialist medical expertise with assistance to be provided by nurses and/or midwives. The latter view has been in the forefront in recent years and has been associated with increased involvement of medical staff in normal maternity care and concomitant constraints on the role that the majority of midwives were once able to fulfil.

The second focus of the debate has been concerned with opportunities for developing and expanding the role of the midwife as patterns and expectations of maternity care change. As Grant (1984) comments, midwives in many countries now seek to provide care and support for women in the context of an ever-increasing complexity of obstetric procedures and investigative techniques, ethical dilemmas posed by developments in reproductive medicine, and consumer expectations that care should be designed to meet the needs and requests of the individual. In particular, attention has focused on the potential benefits of midwifery care and support for certain groups of women; for example, those who are economically or socially disadvantaged, those who have a high-risk pregnancy, and those who experience a perinatal or neonatal death or the birth of a handicapped child (Gilligan, 1980; Social Services Committee, 1980; Newson, 1985; Collins, 1986).

The history of the midwifery profession in Britain has been one of a gradual change in role from an independent practitioner providing care throughout pregnancy, labour and the puerperium, to that of a member of a team of health professionals in which each midwife is likely to be involved in only part of this care (Cowell and Wainwright, 1981; Robinson *et al.*, 1983; Towler and Brammall, 1986). Many have expressed concern that the midwife's skills were not fully utilized within this team, particularly in the provision of care during pregnancy. The Royal College of Midwives, in giving their evidence to the Royal Commission on the National Health Service, expressed this view in their statement that 'The midwife is trained and capable of giving prenatal care on her own responsibility, but in practice the medical staff do not fully utilize this valuable resource' (Royal College of Midwives, 1977). Brain (1979) suggested that during the 1970s, the role of the midwife had contracted, particularly in relation to antenatal care, and that 'in some clinics midwives are only used as receptionists or chaperones and to test urine and weigh women'. In commenting on developments in the 1970s, Barnett (1979) said although midwives regarded doctors as their partners, in her opinion the reverse was not always true. Concern about the erosion of the midwife's role is not, however, purely a British phenomenon. In a recent review of studies of the role of the midwife in developed countries, Barclay (1985) has drawn attention to the consistent finding that midwifery skills are frequently under-utilized, mainly as a consequence of the involvement of medical staff in an increasing proportion of maternity cases. A recent report on perinatal services in 23 European countries also drew attention to this problem (World Health Organisation, 1985).

The study described in this chapter was undertaken in 1979 when concern about the role of the midwife in the United Kingdom was at its height. It comprises an analysis of the role and responsibilities of the midwife, focusing in particular on the degree of responsibility midwives were able to exercise for decision-making and on the interrelationship of these responsibilities with those of medical staff. It was funded by the Department of Health and Social Security and supported from the outset by the Royal College of Midwives and the then Central Midwives' Board.

The data are now nearly ten years old but are included in this volume for two reasons. First, they provide a benchmark for the role of the midwife in the late 1970s, against which findings from subsequent studies on this topic can be compared; a number of such studies will be included in later volumes in this series. Secondly, the study represented a 'broad brush' approach to the subject, in that data on many aspects of the midwife's role were obtained. These aspects included procedures and activities carried out, responsibilities for decision-making in normal antepartum, intrapartum and postpartum care, views on the division of responsibility between midwives and others, views on staffing levels and on continuity of care, career plans and job satisfaction (Robinson, 1980; Robinson *et al.*, 1983; Robinson, 1985a,b,c,d,e,f). The study thus provided some basic information on a wide range of issues relevant to an analysis of the midwife's role, whereas subsequent studies, including some in this volume, have focused on one or more of these topics in greater depth. This chapter focuses in particular on the division of responsibility between midwives and medical staff and on the variation in views held about this division both between and within the two groups.

RESEARCH DESIGN AND FIELDWORK

The research started from the premise that midwives trained in the United Kingdom are qualified to provide women with care throughout pregnancy, labour and the puerperium on their own responsibility and to recognize those deviations from the normal that require referral to medical staff for advice and treatment, that is, in accordance with accepted international definitions of the role of the midwife (World Health Organisation, 1966; International Congress of Midwives/International Federation of Gynaecology and Obstetrics, 1973).

Exploratory work

The initial phase of the research consisted of a series of semi-structured interviews with midwives working in a variety of practice settings and a wide range of other personnel involved in maternity care, as a means of identifying the issues and views current in the late 1970s. These interviews revealed considerable diversity, not only in the level of responsibility exercised by midwives but also in opinions concerning the role they should fulfil in maternity care. In view of this diversity and the paucity of earlier work in the field, a national survey by questionnaire of midwives and the health professionals with whom they are most likely to be working was chosen as the most appropriate method for achieving the aims of the study. A survey on this scale would provide information on the diversity of practice and on overall trends, as well as sufficient numbers of respondents for statistical analysis within subgroups.

Survey design

The survey design was a two-stage random sample stratified by region. One in four of the health districts was selected randomly from each of the 14 Regional Health Authorities and from Wales, providing a total of 60 districts in all. This number was large enough to encompass a wide range of practice situations and provide a large enough sample for subgroup analysis but also small enough to allow time for research access to be negotiated, administrative arrangements to be made and for each district to be visited for delivery of the questionnaires. Personal contact with staff in the course of this visit was regarded as an important factor in encouraging participation in the study, a matter of crucial concern in survey research. The sample sizes required were provided by including all the midwives and medical staff in obstetrics in post in each district, a one in two sample of the health visitors and a one in three sample of general practitioners on the obstetric list in each district.

Piloting questionnaires

Questionnaires covering the topics detailed above were developed and pilot-tested three times in five districts of one Regional Health Authority. Initially, separate questionnaires were drafted for each area in which hospital midwives worked; one for staff in the antenatal clinic, one for staff on the labour ward, and so on. However, having arranged to discuss the antenatal clinic questionnaire, we sometimes discovered that the midwife in question had worked in the labour ward for the last year and had only been in the antenatal clinic for a few weeks. Consequently, she was not given the opportunity to discuss her labour ward experience. Accurate analysis of the midwife's role required information based on an up-to-date experience of a reasonable length. Consequently, a generic questionnaire was designed for all hospital midwives containing a section on each clinical area. Respondents were asked to complete those sections for the areas in which they were currently working or had worked for at least two months in the last two years in their present hospital. They were asked to answer only in relation to experience in their present hospital, so that we could determine the extent to which experience might vary from one type of hospital to another. As the work of community midwives is likely to include all aspects of maternity care, they were asked to complete all sections of their questionnaire.

Interviewing, observation and validity

We decided to interview a sample of the questionnaire respondents so that certain topics could be explored in more depth than was possible by means of questionnaires, for example, midwives' feelings about the division of responsibility, both actual and desired, between different groups.

Attempts to ensure validity of the questionnaire data were of two kinds: first, extensive piloting of the questionnaires as described; secondly, observation of a subsample of respondents who had completed pilot questionnaires and/or participated in interview schedule piloting. The latter procedure, described as between-method triangulation (Denzin, 1978), indicated whether data obtained by different methods produce the same findings (in this case, do midwives do what they say they do?). Details of the methods and instruments used in interviewing and observation can be found in Robinson *et al.* (1983). Data obtained from questionnaires, interviews and observations revealed a high degree of concordance and so it was concluded that the questionnaire satisfied the criteria of validity as well as those of representativeness and reliability.

Main fieldwork

Questionnaires. Questionnaires for midwives and health visitors were delivered personally to managers in each of the 60 districts. The general practitioners' questionnaires were posted to their surgery address and those for medical staff in obstetrics to the hospital at which they worked. The day before the latter were posted, the list of staff in post was checked so that changes in personnel that had occurred since the list was obtained could be taken into account.

Various strategies were employed to encourage a high response rate: handouts about the project were made widely available in each district; letters were sent to secretaries of local branches of the Royal College of Midwives; heads of service were asked to discuss the project at unit meetings; and members of the research team spoke at meetings, study days and refresher courses in many parts of the country. Follow-up letters were sent four to five weeks after the initial posting and had a substantial effect on the final response rates as shown in Table 2.1.

The 4248 midwives who returned a questionnaire represented 19% of those in practice at the time of the survey (Central Midwives Board, 1980). The disappointingly low rate achieved for medical staff in obstetrics was primarily due to a poor response from senior house officers; 46% of this group returned a questionnaire as compared with 57% of senior registrars and 66% of consultants. In this chapter, figures given for all medical staff do not include those from senior house officers as their response rate was regarded as too low to be representative. In cases where data from this group were thought to be of particular interest, they are presented separately but need to be regarded with

Table 2.1 Questionnaire survey response rates

Group	Total number of questionnaires sent out	Response rate before reminders sent out		Response rate after reminders sent out	
		%	no.	%	no.
Midwives	5416	62.0	3359	78.4	4248
Health visitors	1326	74.9	993	88.8	1177
General practitioners on the obstetric list	1849	55.7	1030	66.6	1232
Medical staff in obstetrics	609	39.4	240	54.7	333

Source: Compiled by the author.

caution. The test for differences between proportions was used in the analysis of the data from the four groups (Armitage, 1971); given the large size of the samples involved, the lowest level of significance accepted was $p < 0.001$ unless otherwise stated. A total of 74 midwives were interviewed, drawn randomly from those who had returned a questionnaire in five of the 60 districts.

In this chapter questionnaire data only are presented; a report on the interview data is available in Robinson *et al.* (1983).

MIDWIFERY AND MEDICAL RESPONSIBILITIES FOR ANTEPARTUM CARE

In the late 1970s, many aspects of the role of the midwife were the subject of concern, but it was the antenatal period in particular where opportunities for the midwife to use her skills fully and to exercise her clinical judgement were thought to have been eroded (e.g. Royal College of Midwives, 1977; Brain, 1979).

The majority of midwives who took part in this study said that they carried out the various tasks that constitute normal antenatal care: the initial booking, clinical procedures to assess the growth and development of the fetus and to screen the woman for signs of hypertension, abnormal weight gain and abnormal constituents in the urine, and providing advice. This in itself, however, is not necessarily an indication that they are required to use their clinical judgement in interpreting the findings of the various investigations and in deciding whether a pregnancy is progressing normally.

The study therefore examined in detail the division of responsibility for the two tasks requiring the greatest degree of clinical judgement: the initial booking including interviewing the woman (but excluding the assessment of general health) and the abdominal examination. It is when this latter task is performed and results of all the other routine investigations are available, that the overall assessment of the course of pregnancy is made. Data were obtained on the views of midwives and medical staff as to which members of staff were appropriate to carry out these two tasks in normal cases and who actually undertook them.

Views of members of staff appropriate to carry out initial interviews and abdominal examination

The views of hospital and community midwives, medical staff in obstetrics, and general practitioners as to which members of staff they regarded as appropriate to carry out the initial interview and the abdominal examination are shown in Table 2.2 and reveal a considerable disparity.

The data show that hospital and community midwives were much more likely to regard themselves, rather than medical staff, as appropriate to carry out the initial booking. Both differences shown are significant at

Table 2.2 Proportion of respondents who said midwife was appropriate member of staff to carry out initial booking and abdominal examination in normal cases and proportion who said doctor was appropriate member of staff to carry out these tasks

(1) Carrying out the initial booking including interviewing woman and recording history

Group of respondents	Percentage who said:		
	Midwife *is appropriate to carry out task* %	Doctor *is appropriate to carry out task*	
		Consultant or registrar %	Senior house officer %
Hospital midwives ($n = 634$)	90.7	40.4	40.1
Consultants ($n = 121$)	75.7	75.2	35.5
Senior registrars ($n = 24$)	50.0	91.7	33.3
Registrars ($n = 65$)	67.7	63.1	30.8
Senior house officers ($n = 113$)	71.6	54.0	44.2
		General practitioner	
Community midwives ($n = 1159$)	87.3	58.2	
General practitioners ($n = 1232$)	47.2	87.4	

the 0.00001 level. The midwives were also more likely to regard themselves, rather than medical staff, as appropriate to carry out the abdominal examination; the differences were not as great as for the initial booking, but still significant at the 0.00001 level. The general practitioners were significantly more likely to regard themslves, rather than community midwives, as appropriate to carry out these two tasks (87.4% compared with 47.2% for the initial booking ($p < 0.00001$) and 92.8% compared with 67.9% for the abdominal examination ($p < 0.00001$). The medical staff in obstetrics were more likely to regard the doctor (consultant, registrar or house officer), rather than the midwife, as appropriate to carry out the abdominal examination. The views of the more junior grades of medical staff are of particular interest in that they were significantly less likely than the senior grades to regard the midwife as appropriate to carry out the abdominal examination. This may be because they have trained at a time when the midwife's responsibility for making antenatal assessments had already diminished.

(2) Carrying out the abdominal examination

Group of respondents	Percentage who said:		
	Midwife *is appropriate to carry out task*	Doctor *is appropriate to carry out task*	
		Consultant or registrar	*Senior house officer*
	%	%	%
Hospital midwives (*n* = 634)	87.9	72.7	74.4
Consultants (*n* = 121)	74.4	88.4	83.5
Senior registrars (*n* = 24)	79.2	91.7	91.7
Registrars (*n* = 65)	58.5	75.4	70.8
Senior house officers (*n* = 113)	51.3	66.4	86.7
		General practitioner	
Community midwives (*n* = 1159)	90.2	75.5	
General practitioners (*n* = 1232)	67.9	92.8	

Source: Compiled by the author.

Data relating to the initial booking show that the medical staff in obstetrics were less likely than the midwives to regard the midwife as appropriate to carry out this task. They were, however, more likely to regard the midwife, rather than the senior house officer, as appropriate in this respect.

Actual responsibility for the initial interview and abdominal examination

Despite the finding that the majority of midwives regarded the midwife as an appropriate member of staff to carry out the two tasks, this was not always translated into practice. Taking the initial interview first, the data in Table 2.3 show that 75% of hospital midwives and 48% of community midwives worked in clinics in which they did carry out this interview. However, 21.3% of hospital midwives and 36.9% of community midwives worked in clinics in which the doctor undertook the interview or repeated it after the midwife had done so.

The situation with regard to the abdominal examination was much more extreme. Although midwives are qualified to interpret the findings of this examination on their own responsibility, the survey revealed that

Table 2.3 Hospital and community midwives' responsibility for the initial interview

Responsibility for interview	Midwives in consultant units		Community midwives	
	%	no.	%	no.
Usually carried out by midwife only	75.4	478	48.3	560
Usually carried out by doctor only	1.3	8	15.4	179
Carried out by midwife but usually repeated by doctor	20.0	127	21.5	249
Carried out by midwife at one visit and by doctor at next	–	–	5.4	63
Situation varies from one clinic to another	–	–	7.3	85
No answer	3.3	21	2.0	23
Total	100.0	634	100.0	1159

Source: Compiled by the author.

very few in fact worked in clinics in which they were able to do so. This is shown in Table 2.4.

The data in column one show that the great majority of hospital midwives worked in clinics in which medical staff were responsible for the assessment of pregnancy, in that 33.4% said the examination was carried out by a doctor only and 57.3% said it was carried out by a midwife but then repeated by a doctor. It can, of course, be argued that one of the reasons why many women attending hospital antenatal clinics are always examined by a doctor is that with the advent of 'shared' antenatal care with the general practitioner, visits to the hospital clinic are regarded as being for the specific purpose of assessment by the obstetrician. However, the data in the second column of Table 2.4 show that when women visit community antenatal clinics they are also likely to be assessed by medical staff, in that 16.7% of the community midwives said the abdominal examination was usually carried out by the doctor only and 48.7% said that it was carried out by the midwife but usually repeated by the doctor. Almost 14% said that they were responsible for the abdominal examin- ation and a further 15.4% said this was the case some of the time. As one community midwife put it, 'The first doctor I work for examines patients completely himself. The second doctor leaves it to me. The third doctor checks.' In total, just under a third of the community midwives were

Table 2.4 Hospital and community midwives' responsibility for abdominal examination

Responsibility for abdominal examination	Midwives in consultant units		Community midwives	
	%	no.	%	no.
Usually carried out by midwife only	4.3	27	13.9	161
Usually carried out by doctor only	33.4	212	16.7	193
Carried out by midwife but usually repeated by doctor	57.3	363	48.7	564
Carried out by midwife at one visit and by doctor at next	–	–	6.8	79
Situation varies from one clinic to another	–	–	8.6	100
No answer	5.0	32	5.3	62
Total	100.0	634	100.0	1159

Source: Complied by the author.

responsible for the abdominal examination in some or all of the clinics in which they worked, but this was the case for less than 5% of the hospital midwives.

In order to establish whether midwives ever had the opportunity to take responsibility for the overall assessment of pregnancy, the midwives and the medical staff were asked: 'Are all patients who attend your antenatal clinic examined by a doctor at every visit?'

The data in Table 2.5 show that a substantial proportion of hospital and community midwives worked in clinics in which they never had the opportunity to rely entirely on their own skills and judgement in assessing the course of pregnancy. The data also show that medical staff in obstetrics were significantly more likely than hospital midwives to indicate that all women were examined by a doctor at every visit ($p < 0.00001$), and that general practitioners were significantly more likely to say that this was the case than midwives participating in clinics held at general practitioners' surgeries ($p < 0.00001$) or midwives participating in clinics held at health centres ($p < 0.00001$).

The lack of opportunity for midwives to use their skills and clinical judgement when working in clinics in which doctors are responsible for

Table 2.5 Midwives and medical staff: proportion who said all women were examined by a doctor at every visit to the clinic

Group of respondents	Respondents in each location who said all women examined by a doctor at every visit	
	%	no.
Hospital Staff		
Midwives ($n = 634$)	43.2	274
Medical staff in obstetrics ($n = 210$)	65.7	138
Community Staff		
Midwives participating in clinics held at general practitioners' surgeries ($n = 802$)	48.3	387
Midwives participating in clinics held at health centres ($n = 384$)	55.2	212
General practitioners who held antenatal sessions in which midwives participated ($n = 803$)	68.2	548

Source: Compiled by the author.

the assessment of pregnancy and the frustration this causes were graphically described by some of the survey respondents.

The midwives "snatch" the chance to examine patients, but the procedure is always repeated by the consultant.

(Staff midwife)

The midwife is trained and capable of performing these tasks. Time would be saved if doctors would respect the midwives' opinions.

(Hospital sister)

Midwives in this unit do everything for the patient with the exception of abdominal examination, and we have to get in quickly with our pupils if we want to teach palpation.

(Staff midwife)

In some of the antenatal clinics I attend the general practitioner insists on repeating the whole antenatal examination as if he distrusts my capabilities and judgement — not very inspiring! In another clinic I examine some of the patients while the general practitioner examines others. I feel he trusts me.

(Community midwifery sister)

The survey data also indicated that few other opportunities existed for midwives to take responsibility for antenatal assessments. Midwives' clinics were held in only 26 of the 71 consultant units included in the survey and in 19 of these only a small proportion of women were seen. As one respondent said:

> There are usually 80–100 patients at a doctor's clinic and 6–12 at a midwives' clinic. It is the doctors who refer patients to the midwives' clinic, not the other way round. I should like this reversed and for the midwife to be responsible for the antenatal care of the normal midwifery patient.

> (Sister)

Community midwives do have the opportunity to monitor a woman's progress when they visit at home during the antenatal period, but the data showed that few home visits were made for this purpose.

These data thus confirmed the concern expressed by midwives about the erosion of their role in the antenatal period. While most of those who took part in this study carried out the various procedures that constitute routine antenatal care, the majority practised in situations in which medical staff and not midwives took the responsibility for deciding whether or not a woman's pregnancy was progressing satisfactorily.

Views of midwives and medical staff on the division of responsibility for antenatal care

How did the respondents – midwives and medical staff – regard this state of affairs? Two questions provided some information on their feelings in this respect: first, views on the division of responsibility between midwives and medical staff, and second, changes wanted in the midwife's role in antenatal care.

Midwives' views. Midwives were asked to indicate which of the options shown in Table 2.6 described their view of the division of responsibility between themselves and medical staff in the antenatal period. The figures in column 1 and column 5 show that nearly 60% of the hospital midwives and 72% of the community midwives thought the division was about right. The antenatal data thus present a confusing picture: nearly all the members of both groups of midwives were shown to regard the midwife as appropriate to carry out the key task of the abdominal examination (Table 2.2) but despite the fact that nearly all the hospital midwives and two-thirds of the community midwives worked in clinics in which doctors and not midwives carried it out (Table 2.4), the majority nonetheless said the division of responsibility with medical staff was about right. When these data were analysed by the respondents' answers to the question on actual responsibility for the abdominal examination (Table 2.4), significant differences emerged among the groups of hospital midwives (Table 2.6) but not among their community colleagues. Thus

Table 2.6 Hospital and community midwives: views on division of responsibility between midwives and medical staff

Views on division of responsibility	All hospital midwives (n = 634)		Hospital midwives working in clinics in which abdominal examinations were:						All community midwives (n = 1159)	
			Usually carried out by midwife (n = 27)		Usually carried out by doctor (n = 212)		Carried out by midwife but usually repeated by doctor (n = 363)			
	%	no.	%	no.	%	no.	%	no.	%	no.
About right	58.7	372	77.8	21	54.7	116	59.0	214	71.6	830
Medical staff are undertaking tasks which should be undertaken by midwives	37.7	239	22.2	6	40.1	85	38.3	139	24.8	287
Midwives are undertaking tasks which should be undertaken by medical staff	15.1	96	14.8	4	9.9	21	17.9	65	13.2	153
No answer	1.1	7	–	–	1.9	4	1.1	4	–	–

Source: Compiled by the author.

N.B. (i) The figures in each column add up to more than 100%, as some respondents ringed both options 2 and 3.
   (ii) 5.0% (32) of the hospital midwives did not answer the question on responsibility for carrying out the abdominal examination and therefore the figures in columns 2, 3 and 4 add up to 602.

78% of hospital midwives who said the abdominal examination was carried out by the midwife also thought that the division of responsibility with medical staff was about right. Although this proportion fell for the two groups who worked in clinics in which the examination was carried out by medical staff, it nevertheless remained a majority at 54.7% and 59.0% respectively.

Most of the comments made by the 37.7% of hospital midwives who thought medical staff were undertaking tasks that should be undertaken by midwives referred to the erosion of the midwife's role in the assessment of pregnancy. For example, a staff midwife said:

> We are adequately experienced to assess a normal pregnancy and palpate abdomens (often more accurately than new house officers). Our main role in clinic is caring for the doctor – not the patient.

When hospital midwives were asked about changes they would like to see in the midwife's role in antenatal care, 47% said they wanted the midwife to have more responsibility for assessment *vis-à-vis* the doctor. In the view of a sister:

> Patients should be seen by the midwife and only referred to the doctor if necessary. This would cut down on waiting times at clinics and give more time for the midwife to listen to the problems of the patient.

Two-thirds of the comments referred specifically to midwives' clinics. In the words of a staff midwife:

> I would like a midwives' clinic – this would be satisfying for the midwife, more leisurely for the patient and provide an excellent teaching opportunity for students.

As shown in Table 2.6, only a quarter of the community midwives felt medical staff were undertaking tasks that should have been undertaken by midwives. All the comments made by this group referred to responsibility for antenatal assessments, some focusing on the way the midwife's role had changed in this respect. As one of them said:

> The full examination of a patient should be undertaken by a midwife, including the abdominal examination, and the patient referred to medical staff if any abnormality arises. We have been reduced to mere chaperones over the last few years.

The community respondents were less likely than their hospital colleagues to say they wanted more responsibility for antenatal assessments (15.3% compared with 47.2%). Those who did referred to the lack of use of the midwife's skills, skills which, as some respondents noted, were once used more fully:

> It would be nice to have more responsibility in the antenatal care of patients. We were taught the skill of palpation, etc. Why can't we use it?

I would like to see a return to the practising midwife taking responsibility for the antenatal care of the normal pregnant woman, referring the illnesses and abnormalities of pregnancy to the obstetrician
— not the GP, unless he is specially trained.

Two-thirds (37) of the heads of midwifery service wanted their staff to
have an increased level of responsibility in this respect, and this is a larger
proportion than that found among the staff they managed, namely 47.2%
of hospital midwives and 15.3% of those working in the community. The
views of the heads of service covered many of the issues raised by the
staff in practice: in particular, the waste of the midwife's skills and the
quality of care provided for women:

The trend is for all patients to be seen by a doctor at every antenatal
visit and I would like to see a return of the midwives' clinic where
patients have more time to discuss problems with the midwives.

I think it's very sad to see midwives who really know what antenatal
care is about having to take second place to junior medical staff . . . .
Midwives have far more experience than any of the junior doctors
do; they pick up the abnormal and know when to refer.

Interestingly, 15 of the 24 heads of service who were satisfied with the
level of responsibility their staff enjoyed said this was because all, or at
least some of the midwives, were able to take full responsibility for antenatal assessments, usually at midwives' clinics.

A diversity of view about the midwife's role had been shown to exist
among the hospital and community staff, and the same was true for the
heads of service. Two members of this latter group, for example, said all
antenatal clinics should be run by doctors, and another said she would
worry that midwives would not know when to refer. The data obtained
from the heads of service raise an important question: as so few midwives
practised in situations in which they were not able to assess the course of
pregnancy on their own responsibility (Table 2.4) and two-thirds of the
heads of service thought midwives should have more responsibility, why
did a situation exist in which the skills of the midwife were wasted in this
way? It was outside the terms of reference of the project reported here to
examine this question in detail. The answer would have to be sought in an
historical analysis, focusing on the way in which changes in the organization and philosophy of antenatal care (Oakley, 1984) had eroded the
midwife's role slowly over a period of years (Cowell and Wainwright,
1981; Robinson *et al.*, 1983), and so became manifest to midwifery
managers gradually rather than at a particular point in time; the former
being less likely to lead to counter-action than the latter. The analysis
would also need to examine the extent to which midwifery managers were
in a position to influence the direction of changes in antenatal care
through representation on relevant committees and decision-making
bodies.

Table 2.7 Obstetricians and general practitioners: views on the division of responsibility between midwives and medical staff in the antenatal period

Views on division of responsibility	Obstetricians: consultants senior registrars, and registrars (n = 210)		General practitioners in practices in which primary health care team includes a midwife (n = 1006)	
	%	no.	%	no.
About right	69.5	146	85.4	859
Medical staff are undertaking tasks which should be undertaken by midwives	23.3	49	11.2	113
Midwives are undertaking tasks which should be undertaken by medical staff	8.1	17	3.8	38
No answer	4.3	9	3.1	31

Source: Compiled by the author.

N.B. The figures in each column add up to more than 100%, as some respondents ringed both options 2 and 3.

The views of medical staff. The views of obstetricians and general practitioners present a much less complex picture than those of the midwives. The majority of both groups, as shown in Table 2.7, regarded the division of responsibility between themselves and midwives in the antenatal period as about right. As data in Table 2.4 indicated, the majority of these doctors would have been working in clinics in which they and not the midwife usually took responsibility for overall antenatal assessments. Further confirmation of the findings that medical staff regard this situation as appropriate came from analysing data on whether all women were examined by a doctor at every visit to the clinic by views on the division of responsibility: 70% of the obstetricians and 80% of the general practitioners who said that all women were examined by a doctor at every visit also said that the division of responsibility between midwives and medical staff was about right.

Some statements of dissent were made, however; 47 of the 49 obstetricians who said that in their view medical staff undertook tasks that should be performed by midwives commented on their questionnaire that midwives should have more responsibility for antenatal care. In the words of a senior registrar:

Midwives are used mainly for performing non-specialised tasks
such as recording blood pressure and weight .... They would be
better employed in performing the majority of antenatal care and
screening out potential problems for medical staff.

Two reasons were proffered by obstetricians as to why it was difficult
to restore responsibility for assessing pregnancy to midwives. The first
consideration was the training needs of junior doctors:

Midwives are quite capable of doing more of the routine antenatal
examinations, but in order to train house officers in antenatal care,
it is necessary for them to do the routine palpations.

(Consultant)

The second reason given was that midwives now lacked the confidence to
run their own clinics.

MIDWIFERY AND MEDICAL RESPONSIBILITIES FOR INTRAPARTUM CARE

Investigating the division of responsibility between midwives and medical
staff for the care of women during labour and delivery was more complex
than the corresponding division of responsibility for antepartum care.

In the latter instance it was known that the midwife's role had been
restricted because doctors were now carrying out the tasks once regarded
as the province of the midwife and the data in the preceding section
demonstrated the extent to which this was the case in England and Wales
in 1979. Although the incidence of operative and instrumental deliveries
increased during the 1970s, the midwife continued to be the most senior
person present at the majority of deliveries (Chamberlain *et al.*, 1978,
Cartwright, 1979). However, as Oakley (1976) comments, these statistics
may demonstrate the continuing importance of the midwife, but they are
uninformative about her degree of autonomy within the reproductive care
system.

During the 1970s, medical staff assumed a greater role in the assessment and management of normal labour than before. This was primarily
through the formulation of unit policies specifying the nature of procedures to be followed, such as the frequency of vaginal examinations, the
length of time to be allowed for the second stage of labour and whether
or not to use continuous fetal heart rate monitoring. Consequently, this
research sought to ascertain the extent of the midwife's autonomy in clinical decision-making in the care of women during labour and delivery in
this increasingly medicalized context.

Midwives and obstetricians were asked which of the situations
described in Table 2.8 usually applied in the labour ward in which they
worked. Two main points emerge from the data: first, a substantial
majority of midwives said that women in normal labour are cared for by a
midwife and only examined by a doctor at a midwife's request; secondly,

Table 2.8 Midwives and obstetricians: management of normal labour

Management of normal labour	Midwives in consultant units		Medical staff in obstetrics	
	%	*no.*	%	*no.*
Patients in normal labour are cared for by a midwife and only examined by a doctor if this is requested by a midwife	79.8	1260	45.7	96
All patients are examined by a doctor on admission and then normal labours are managed entirely by a midwife unless a problem arises	11.7	185	28.1	59
All patients are examined by a doctor on admission, visited at regular intervals throughout labour and the decisions as to management of labour are made by a doctor	4.6	73	22.4	47
No answer	3.9	61	3.8	8
Total	100.0	1579	100.0	210

Source: Compiled by the author.

the obstetricians were significantly less likely than the midwives to say this was the case (45.7% compared with 79.8% – $p < 0.00001$) and much more likely to indicate that medical staff were involved in the care of women whose labour progressed normally.

As with data on antenatal care, it was not possible in the course of this research to determine whether the perceptions of medical staff were more or less accurate than those of the midwives. Whatever the truth of the matter, however, it is of interest that the perceptions of the two groups of their own responsibilities for the care of women in labour differed so greatly. As noted on page 12, data from senior house officers are not included in the medical staff figures because of the low response rate, but it is worthy of note that of the 46% of staff in this grade who did return a questionnaire, 79% selected the first option shown in Table 2.8. This percentage differed significantly from that of their senior colleagues ($p <$ 0.00001) but not from that of midwives.

Midwives may be exercising their clinical judgement when making decisions concerning the care of women in normal labour, or they may be required to follow a unit policy or a decision made by a doctor with regard to some aspects of this care. The figures in Table 2.8 show that a total of 1445 of the midwives said they worked in units in which normal labours were managed by the midwife. In order to ascertain the proportion who worked in units in which aspects of this management were determined by unit policy or medical decisions, midwives were asked who was responsible for the decisions listed in Table 2.9.

The data on decision-making show that by 1979 the midwife's freedom to make decisions basic to the care of women in normal labour had to some extent been curtailed. The proportion of respondents who said the midwife made the decision varied from one procedure to another: from 36.9% for using continuous fetal heart rate monitoring machines to 94.3% for carrying out an episiotomy. Just under half of the respondents said the frequency with which vaginal examinations were carried out was determined by unit policy and a substantial minority said this was the case for rupturing membranes, using continuous fetal heart rate monitoring machines and giving intramuscular analgesics.

The 155 obstetricians who had said the midwife managed normal labour were also asked the question about responsibility for specific decisions. They were significantly less likely than midwives to say the midwife made the decisions, as shown in Table 2.10 (the level of significance ranged from $p < 0.001$ for vaginal examination to $p < 0.00001$ for using continuous fetal heart rate monitoring machines). Thus the data again revealed contrasting perceptions of the relative responsibilities held by midwives and obstetricians.

There was in fact some evidence from this study that midwives may overestimate the extent to which they make decisions based on their own clinical judgement and underestimate the extent to which they practise according to prevailing unit policies. Thus in response to a question concerning the frequency with which certain obstetric procedures were carried out in the labour ward in which they worked, 374 midwives said episiotomies were performed too often; however, 92% of this group also said that it was the midwife who made the decision whether or not to perform an episiotomy. It is unlikely that midwives would say that a procedure that they decided to carry out was performed too often and more likely that the decision was in fact determined by a unit policy or a medical decision. A similar finding was obtained by Henderson (1984) who demonstrated that midwives underestimate the extent to which decisions to rupture membranes are determined by unit policies or

Table 2.9 Midwives in consultant units: responsibility for decision-making in normal labour

Responsibility for decision-making	Decisions made in the management of normal labour									
	When to carry out vaginal examinations		At what point during labour to rupture membranes		Whether to give intramuscular analgesics		Whether to carry out an episiotomy		Whether to use a continuous monitoring machine	
	%	no.	%	no.	%	no.	%	no.	%	no.
Decision is usually made by a midwife	47.4	685	56.3	814	79.4	1147	94.3	1363	36.9	533
Decision is usually made by a member of the medical staff	0.3	5	10.2	147	2.0	29	0.3	4	30.2	437
There is a unit policy which specifies the usual procedure to be followed	49.3	713	29.7	429	15.5	224	3.2	46	28.2	408
No answer	2.9	42	3.8	55	3.1	45	2.2	32	4.6	67
Total	100.0	1445	100.0	1445	100.0	1445	100.0	1445	100.0	1445

Source: Compiled by the author.

Table 2.10 Hospital midwives and obstetricians: Proportion who said midwife made decisions about management of normal labour

Decision	Midwives in consultants units (n = 1445)		Medical staff in obstetrics (n = 155)	
	%	no.	%	no.
When to carry out vaginal examinations in normal labour	47.4	685	32.9	51
At what point during a normal labour to rupture membranes	56.3	814	30.3	47
Whether to give intra-muscular analgesics in normal labour	79.4	1147	65.8	102
Whether to use a continuous monitoring machine in normal labour	36.9	533	11.6	18
Whether to do an episiotomy	94.3	1363	72.3	112

Source: Compiled by the author.

doctors' decisions and overestimate the extent to which they are made by midwives. Only a small percentage of midwives (6.4%) expressed concern about restrictions on midwives' decision-making. As the following comments show, their concerns focused on loss of skill and the development of judgement by student and recently qualified midwives.

> As the unit policy for procedures is determined by medical staff, the decisions made by midwives are diminishing rapidly. Until quite recently, decisions on vaginal examinations, rupturing membranes, intramuscular analgesics, monitoring and episiotomies would have been the midwife's decision.
>
> (Sister)

> I feel that the role of the midwife is being eroded and that special skills are being lost. Patients are not allowed to labour normally nowadays. Therefore decision-making by the midwife is a disappearing art.
>
> (Sister)

> In the hospital where I work, the midwives who have qualified

longer take much more initiative whereas newly trained midwives are inclined to let decisions be made by the medical staff.

(Sister)

Unit policy states that all primips must have an episiotomy. In some primips they are totally unnecessary, but students qualify without having delivered a primip with an intact perineum and never develop any judgement of their own.

(Sister)

In summary, the data on the midwife's role in the care of women during normal labour and delivery in hospital show that the majority of midwives perceived that they were responsible for this care; albeit that some of them also said that aspects of this care were determined by unit policies or medical decisions. Medical staff, on the other hand, were significantly less likely than midwives to attribute this degree of responsibility to the midwife.

How satisfied were hospital midwives and medical staff with the division of responsibility they perceived as existing between them for the care of women during normal labour and delivery? Seventy-five percent of both groups in fact said it was 'about right' and few dissenting voices were raised. The 21% of midwives who felt medical staff were undertaking tasks that were the midwife's responsibility either referred to their desire to suture, set up intravenous infusions, and so on, or said that medical staff intervened too much in the management of normal labour. In the words of a sister:

Vaginal examinations in normal labour could be done by a midwife, but the doctors carry on and do them. Doctors are present at normal labours telling patients when to push and telling the midwife when to do an episiotomy.

Comments made by medical staff also reflected these two themes: namely, midwives taking on technical procedures such as suturing and the question of responsibility for managing labour. In the latter regard, some obstetricians regretted that midwives enjoyed less responsibility than previously.

At present doctors have taken over much of the traditional role of the midwife. The modern midwife has been brainwashed to give up much more of her responsibility to the doctor. The midwifery hierarchy are to blame for this.

(Consultant)

The present trend for doctors to control labour in normal cases should be reversed.

(Senior Registrar)

Others, usually more junior staff, expressed the opposite view. Thus:

All patients should be seen by medical staff on admission and regularly throughout labour. Doctors should not only attend the labour

ward when requested but should *dictate* the management of labour.
[respondent's emphasis]

(Registrar)

Unit policies should be made by the obstetrician in charge and be
strictly adhered to by the midwife.

(Registrar)

Community midwives' responsibilities for caring for women during labour and delivery

The policy that confinements should take place in a consultant obstetric
unit has led to a continuing decline in the number of deliveries undertaken by community midwives. Figures published by the Central
Midwives Board show that the average number of home deliveries undertaken was 55.3 per midwife in 1959, but by 1979 had fallen to 3.1
(Central Midwives Board, 1960 and 1980). Forty-five percent of the
midwives who participated in this survey had not undertaken any home
deliveries in the last complete year before the research was undertaken,
and of those who had done so, the majority had carried out five or fewer.
When respondents were asked if they were willing to undertake
home confinements, 56% said they were willing to do so in low-risk
cases, while 29% said they were willing only if a patient particularly
insisted and 9% said they would refuse under any circumstances. The
heads of midwifery service were fairly evenly divided in their views; half
said they were in favour of home confinements and half said they were
opposed to them. When the community midwives were asked what
factors prevented them from booking women for home confinements,
views of other health professionals featured prominently in that 64%
cited the reluctance of general practitioners to provide medical cover, and
33% cited a local policy of opposition to home confinements.

Turning to the views of medical staff themselves, 75% of the general
practitioners said it was the policy of their practice to discourage or
oppose home confinements and 82% of the obstetricians said that they
were not in favour of home deliveries, even for women with an anticipated
low-risk pregnancy.

Since the late 1960s, community midwives have been able to deliver
some women in hospital, with the creation of schemes such as the
'domino' system (whereby community midwives care for women in the
antenatal period, deliver them in hospital, take them home within 24
hours and care for them in the community during the postnatal period).
Figures published by the Central Midwives Board show that the number
of women delivered in hospital by community midwives has risen from
five per midwife in 1972 to eight per midwife in 1979 (Central Midwives
Board, 1973 and 1980). When the midwives who took part in this study
were asked about their involvement in domino schemes, 76% said that
they had not undertaken any domino deliveries in the year preceding the

survey. Of those who had, the majority had undertaken fewer than ten. Fifty-eight percent of the community midwives said they were in favour of extending the domino scheme to a greater number of women in their district, and this proportion rose to 81% among those who had actually undertaken domino deliveries. Reasons given by midwives as to why it was difficult to extend the scheme included distances from the maternity unit, shortages of midwives and reluctance on the part of general practitioners to book women for this type of delivery.

Whether or not such schemes do become more widely available depends to a large extent on the views of medical staff. Fifty-seven per cent of the general practitioners who took part in this survey said they were in favour of domino schemes. Reasons such as continuity of care for the mother, job satisfaction for the midwife and a good compromise between home and hospital confinement were cited for holding this view. Fifty-six per cent of the medical staff in obstetrics said they were in favour of domino deliveries for women with low-risk pregnancies, although one-fifth of this group added a proviso that responsibility for management of the patients should remain with the consultant. Reasons given by the medical staff who were opposed to domino deliveries included distances from the maternity unit, a shortage of midwives, the need for all deliveries to be carried out under medical supervision and community midwives lacking sufficient delivery experience and familiarity with hospital labour ward technology.

MIDWIFERY AND MEDICAL RESPONSIBILITIES FOR POSTPARTUM CARE

Medical involvement in normal postnatal care is not usually an issue for community midwives as they provide this on their own responsibility in the woman's home, calling in medical staff if necessary. It is an issue, however, in the hospital context. Data on clinical assessment of normal women after delivery obtained in the course of this study demonstrated a duplication of midwifery and medical roles similar to that found in assessment during pregnancy. Midwives are qualified to assess the condition of the postpartum woman and make daily examinations to do so. The majority participating in this study, however, worked in consultant units in which medical staff also examined normal postnatal women, either once or twice during their stay (55%), or daily (26%). Only 17% of respondents said medical staff examined normal postnatal women only if asked to do so by a midwife. Additionally, over 80% of midwives worked in units in which medical staff always made the decision as to whether the woman and her baby were fit to go home – a decision that midwives are also qualified to make. Many respondents commented that it was more appropriate for this decision to be made by the midwifery team than by the medical team since the former provided continuous care after delivery and were thus in a better position than the latter to assess accurately whether women were emotionally and physically ready for discharge.

Despite the finding that medical staff were involved to some considerable extent in normal postnatal care, the majority of midwives (85%) felt this division of responsibility to be 'about right'. Only 87 comments were made to the effect that midwives' responsibilities in the postpartum period were being eroded. Not surprisingly perhaps, 86% of the medical staff pronounced themselves satisfied with the division of responsibility between themselves and midwives for postnatal care.

IMPLICATIONS OF THE FINDINGS

The research described in this chapter demonstrated that although midwives carried out a major part of the care provided for childbearing women, a substantial proportion were not required to exercise fully the degree of clinical responsibility for which they were trained and qualified, as they worked in situations in which medical staff had assumed this responsibility. The study therefore confirmed the concerns of the profession that the midwife's role was being eroded.

These constraints on the midwife's responsibilities for normal maternity care raise important implications for the maternity services. First, the underuse of midwifery knowledge and skills wastes resources. Midwives are trained at some considerable cost, but once qualified, those parts of their training that concern decision-making, particularly in the assessment of pregnancy, are likely to be wasted. The repetition by medical staff of procedures that have been carried out by midwives and that midwives are qualified to carry out on their own responsibility duplicates resources. Community antenatal care is a particular case in point. Midwives are specifically trained to provide care for women with a low-risk pregnancy, paid a salary to do so, and yet many general practitioners are also paid to provide care for the same group of women.

Secondly, the medical take-over of decision-making for normal pregnancy, labour and the puerperium limits opportunities for students to develop confidence in their skills and decision-making ability and limits opportunities for qualified midwives to maintain their confidence. As shown in this chapter, many of the survey respondents commented to this effect. Unit policies, whether formulated by medical staff alone or by medical staff in consultation with senior midwives, restrict the development and maintenance of clinical judgement and require midwives to follow predetermined courses of action, whether or not they regard it as appropriate in particular cases. This in turn may lead to problems when policies change if the necessary skills have been lost with the retirement of experienced midwives and have not been developed in more recently trained practitioners.

Thirdly, the research demonstrated wide variation in the degree of responsibility midwives were able to exercise and this in turn creates difficulties in the development of appropriate curricula for midwifery training. If training is designed to enable midwives to assume a particular level of responsibility, then many are likely to experience the frustration and lack of job satisfaction that results from unfulfilled expectations.

Finally, and most importantly, the data from this study have a number of implications for the quality of care available to women. Failure to make full use of the clinical skills and judgement of the midwife also affects the kind of support they are able to provide. Thus when medical staff undertake the assessment of normal pregnancy, care is likely to fragment into a number of tasks undertaken by different personnel – doctors and midwives, and in some clinics, nursing and auxiliary staff as well. This fragmentation, combined with the large number of women often attending clinics, means that each woman has only brief contact with each person involved in her care. In this situation midwives have neither time nor opportunity to develop the kind of supportive and continuous relationship within which women feel encouraged to discuss their pregnancy and voice their problems or concerns. Medical involvement in the care of all pregnant women also contributes to long waiting times. Complaints about both these factors, lack of opportunity for discussion and long periods of waiting, feature prominently in consumers' view of antenatal care (National Childbirth Trust, 1981; Garcia, 1982) and were of concern to many of the midwives who took part in this study. As one of the sisters said:

> We need more time to talk to patients, especially those whose first visit it is. The first visit is, I think, very important and so often the patients are rushed around and you can't get to know them or they are so flustered and nervous they forget to ask questions.

A staff midwife commented:

> We need more complete care of individual patients, rather than taking blood pressures, directing pregnant bodies on and off couches so that there is always one 'prepared' and the doctor does not lose precious seconds as he rushes from one to the next.

In these situations also, medical staff have less time to spend with those women who do require specialist medical and obstetric expertise.

It can be argued that if midwives are not entrusted with the care of normal pregnant women, a role for which they are qualified, then they may lose confidence in their own ability and become less able to increase the confidence of pregnant women who look to them for support. Cartwright's (1979) study demonstrated that many women felt they were given insufficient information during the course of labour. This point has been further explored by Kirkham (see Chapter 6), who concluded that one of the reasons midwives fail to provide women with information during labour is that they themselves are unhappy with the policies they are required to implement in the mangement of their care.

In the period since this research was completed, many of the findings have been substantiated by other studies (DHSS, 1984; Garcia *et al.*, 1985; volume 2 of this series). Practising midwives, representatives of statutory and professional bodies and parliamentry committees have expressed their concern at the continued underuse of the midwife's skills; see for example Social Services Committee (1980), Maclean (1980), Fisher (1981), Morrin (1982), Towler (1982), Roch (1983), Central Midwives Board for Scotland *et al.* (1983) and Ashton (1987).

OPTIONS FOR THE FUTURE

Does it matter that midwifery skills and knowledge are wasted in this way, and that decision-making has increasingly been concentrated in the hands of medical staff? Randomized controlled trials that have compared the outcomes when women are cared for primarily by midwives with those when women are cared for primarily by medical staff have in fact demonstrated that midwives achieve neonatal and perinatal outcomes as satisfactory as those achieved by medical staff, while at the same time women in the care of midwives are less likely to require pain control and to experience an operative delivery (Runnerstrom, 1969; Slome *et al.*, 1976; Flint and Poulengeris, 1987). A number of retrospective studies from North America that compared midwifery with medical care have also demonstrated the excellent results achieved by nurse midwives (see, for example, Levy *et al.*, 1971; Dillon *et al.*, 1978; Raisler, 1985; Thompson, 1986).

There is thus no evidence to date that medical staff provide better care than midwives for women with a low-risk pregnancy. The restriction of the midwife's role, however, not only deprives women of their skills in clinical assessment and monitoring, but is also detrimental to midwives' confidence and to the quality of support they can provide for women in their care. A number of studies have in fact shown how much women appreciate support and information provided by midwives (see, for example, Morgan *et al.*, 1984; Humphrey, 1985; Williams *et al.*, 1985).

Since 1979, when the research described in this chapter was undertaken, a number of government and professional reports have recommended that the midwife's skills should be used more fully, particularly in the care of women with a normal pregnancy (Social Services Committee, 1980; Royal College of Obstetricians and Gynaecologists, 1982; Maternity Services Advisory Committee, 1982; Royal College of Midwives, 1987).

Many midwives have in fact sought to restore their role by setting up schemes in which their skills are appropriately deployed in meeting women's needs. Midwives' clinics have been established (Morrin, 1982; Flint, 1982; Stuart and Judge, 1984) and within some consultant units intrapartum care for low-risk women is provided by midwives (Towler, 1981; Rider, 1983; Curran, 1986; Flint and Poulengeris, 1987). Schemes to help women with particular needs have also been established by midwives; these include antenatal day wards for women not able to stay in hospital (Penny, 1986) and support schemes for parents of preterm babies (Goodley, 1986; Hughes, 1986) and for those who experience a perinatal or neonatal loss (Gilligan, 1980; Mulkerrins and Gunn, 1985;

Collins, 1986). Experimental schemes to assess the effect of midwifery support in pregnancy for women in high-risk categories have been undertaken by midwives working in conjunction with colleagues from other disciplines (see Davies and Evans, in volume 2 of this series; Oakley and Elborne, in press). A particularly important development for the profession has been the implementation of schemes in which small teams of midwives provide continuity of care for women from early pregnancy to the end of the puerperium (Curran, 1986; Flint and Poulengeris, 1987; volume 2 of this series).

What factors hinder or prevent midwives from fulfilling the role for which they are qualified and from being accorded a central place in the provision of maternity care? First, the continuing emphasis on the potential abnormalities of childbirth enhances the role of the obstetric specialist at the expense of the role of the midwife as the practitioner of normal midwifery. There is no dispute that the obstetrican should be responsible for overall clinical management of women with medical or obstetric complications, but there is a lack of clarity as to how much responsibility the obstetrican should have for the care of those women who experience a normal pregnancy, labour and puerperium and how much of this care should be provided by midwives acting on their own responsibility. Secondly, the increasing tendency to see responsibilities for maternity care in terms of the relative roles of the consultant obstetrician on the one hand, and the general practitioner on the other, similarly diminishes the role of the midwife.

Thus with the system of 'shared antenatal care' now commonplace, the care of high-risk women is assigned to the obstetrician and that of low-risk women to the general practitioner with intermittent assessment by the obstetrician. Both the consultant and the general practitioner may decide to delegate responsibility for the antenatal assessments of these women to the midwife, or they may decide to undertake all these assessments themselves. The system of shared care divides the responsibility for the assessment of women with normal pregnancies between two groups of medical staff, yet the midwife is specifically trained to provide care for this group of women. It has recently been suggested that more general practitioners should be involved in the care of low-risk women during labour by increasing the number of general practitioner beds within or adjacent to specialist units in all districts, to enable 'a substantial number of women to be cared for in labour by general practitioners with specialist assistance readily available' (Royal College of Obstetricians and Gynaecologists/Royal College of General Practitioners, 1981). However, it is these low-risk women for whom the midwife is trained to care, and it can be argued that if schemes are implemented whereby more general practitioners are involved in the care of these women, then the same duplication of resources will result as demonstrated in relation to antenatal care.

With regard to midwives and general practitioners, it can be argued that there is an inherent duplication of resources in the system of maternity care in Britain. We train a body of professionals – midwives – to provide clinical care, advice and support for normal childbearing women, and yet, at the same time, assign much of this care to general practitioners.

Another important aspect of the interrelationship between the roles of midwives and medical staff is that of women's access to a midwife. Prior to the introduction of the National Health Service, the community midwife was the first point of contact with the maternity services for the majority of women. Once the new service had been introduced in 1948, an increasing number of general practitioners became involved in maternity care. At the same time, the fact that women could book a general practitioner for delivery without payment of a fee led to a trend in which women went to a general practitioner rather than to a midwife for confirmation of pregnancy (Bent, 1982). Increasingly, the general practitioner and not the midwife became the first point of contact with the maternity services.

In recent years, a number of reports have questioned a system that 'makes the general practitioner the gate-keeper to all other health care services' (Clark, 1984). In the context of maternity care, concern has been expressed for women who are not registered with a general practitioner or who are reluctant to report their pregnancy in the first instance to a doctor. According to the Acheson report on primary health care in inner London, up to 30% of people in some areas are not registered with a general practitioner (London Health Care Planning Consortium, 1981). The report of the Social Services Committee on perinatal and neonatal mortality remarked that it is often the women who are in greatest need of early antenatal care, the socially disadvantaged and the homeless in particular, who have no general practitioner or for whom the present system of reporting pregnancy to a doctor may act as a disincentive to receive early care (Social Services Committee, 1980).

The data demonstrated that medical staff were significantly less likely than midwives to indicate that midwives were responsible for decision-making in normal antepartum and intrapartum care. As already noted it was not possible in the course of this project to ascertain which groups' perceptions were more accurate. However, it was also found that the majority of those medical staff who did not perceive midwives as responsible for decision-making also said that the division of responsibility between themselves and midwives was about right. Consequently, those who attempt to reverse the erosion of the midwife's role, as documented by this study, may well find themselves opposed by members of the medical profession.

What responsibility have midwives themselves had for the kind of restrictions on their role which the survey demonstrated? Views expressed by those who took part revealed a diversity of views: some saw the midwife as a victim of circumstance, unable to prevent the medical take-over, whereas others held the midwife responsible.

Given the degree to which the midwife's skills were wasted and/or duplicated, particularly in the antepartum and postpartum periods, it was perhaps surprising that greater levels of dissatisfaction were not expressed. There was some evidence from the study that the proportion of midwives who felt the division of responsibility with medical staff was 'about right' increased with age-group (Robinson *et al.*, 1983). This could partly but not entirely be attributable to the fact that older midwives tended to work in separate general practitioner units in which midwives enjoyed a greater degree of clinical freedom than their colleagues in consultant units (Robinson, 1985b). The explanation may also be that midwives who are not happy with their role leave the profession; thus those who remain are those who are more willing to accept the restrictions of their role that have characterized developments in the maternity services over the last two decades. This possibility is currently under investigation in the course of a longitudinal study of career patterns of midwives, the findings of which will be reported in volume 3 of this series.

To conclude, there is no evidence to date that any advantages accrue from providing women who experience a normal pregnancy and childbirth with medical as opposed to midwifery care. At the same time, the underuse of midwifery skills has serious implications for the maternity services in terms of wasted resources, loss of expertise, and poorer care for women, particularly in terms of emotional support. Clearly there can be no justification for diminishing the midwife's responsibilities for normal antepartum, intrapartum and postpartum care and, as noted, many midwives have sought to restore their role in this respect.

The argument that childbirth is only 'normal in retrospect' should not be used to deprive midwives of their role in maternity care, nor to deprive women of the benefits of midwifery care. Medical staff are of course needed to provide treatment and advice in the case of deviations from the normal but a doctor is not needed to detect such deviations in the first instance – midwives are qualified to do this and can then refer to medical colleagues as and when appropriate. There is in fact some evidence that midwives are more likely than medical staff to detect complications in pregnancy (Chng *et al.*, 1980).

Those responsible for the organization of the maternity services, including midwifery managers, should ensure that the midwife has a central role in that organization, providing normal maternity care on her own responsibility.

Women who wish to have direct access to a midwife without necessarily seeing a general practitioner first, should be able to do so via local antenatal clinics; the establishment of such clinics has been recommended by the Social Services Committee (1980), the Maternity Services Advisory Committee (1982) and the Royal College of Midwives and Health Visitors Association (1982). This would redress the present imbalance of maternity care at the primary level, which focuses on general practitioners in a way that duplicates resources for some women and at the same time fails to reach others.

As noted, a number of schemes have been suggested, and in some cases implemented, which fully use the midwife's skills in the antenatal period and during labour and the puerperium as well. Midwives in many more areas need to implement and evaluate such schemes, as the needs of childbearing women are best met when midwives can use all their skills: clinical assessment and monitoring, and the provision of advice and emotional support.

ACKNOWLEDGEMENTS

I should like to thank the following: Josephine Golden and Susan Bradley, who worked with me on the study on which this chapter is based; the Department of Health and Social Security, who funded the study; Keith Jacka for computing and statistical assistance; Bea Ogilvie for secretarial assistance; and last but not least, all the midwives, doctors, and health visitors who completed our questionnaires.

REFERENCES

Armitage, P.O. (1971) *Statistical methods in medical research.* Blackwell, Oxford.

Ashton, R. (1987) Interview with Ruth Ashton, General Secretary, Royal College of Midwives. *Midwife Health Visitor and Community Nurse, 23,* (7), 292–300.

Barclay, L. (1985) Australian midwifery training and practice. *Midwifery, 1,* (2), 86–96.

Barnett, Z. (1979) The changing pattern of maternity care and the future role of the midwife. *Midwives Chronicle and Nursing Notes, 92* (1102), 381–84.

Bent, E.A. (1982) The growth and development of midwifery. In Allan, P. and Jolley, M. (eds), *Nursing, midwifery and health visiting since 1900.* Faber and Faber, London.

Brain, M. (1979) Observations of a midwife. Report of a day conference on the reduction of perinatal mortality and morbidity. Children's Committee and Department of Health and Social Security. HMSO, London.

Cartwright, A. (1979) *The dignity of labour.* Tavistock, London.

Central Midwives Board (1960, 1973, and 1980) *Annual reports.* Hymns Ancient and Modern Limited, Suffolk.

Central Midwives Board for Scotland, Northern Ireland Council for Nurses and Midwives, An Bord Altranais, Central Midwives Board (1983) *The role of the midwife.* Hymns Ancient and Modern Limited, Suffolk.

Chamberlain, G., Philipp, E., Howlett, B. and Master, K. (1978) British Births 1970. Vol. 2, *Obstetric care.* William Heinemann Medical Books, London.

Chng, P., Hall, M. and MacGillivray, I. (1980) An audit of antenatal care: the value of the first antenatal visit. *British Medical Journal, 281,* 1184–86.

Clark, J. (1984) Opportunity knocks for primary health care nursing at long last. *Nursing Standard, 354,* 5.

Collins, M. (1986) Care for families following stillbirth and first week deaths. *Midwives Chronicle, 99,* (1176), Supplement, xiii–xv.

Cowell, B. and Wainwright, D. (1981) *Behind the blue door. The history of the Royal College of Midwives, 1881–1981.* Balliere Tindall, London.

Curran, V. (1986) Taking midwifery off the conveyor belt. *Nursing Times* (August 20th, 1986), 42–43.

Denzin, N.K. (1978) *Sociological Methods. A sourcebook. Second edition.* McGraw Hill, New York.

Department of Health and Social Security (1984) Study of hospital based midwives: A report by Central Management Services. Department of Health and Social Security, London.

Dillon, T., Brennan, B., Dwyer, Y., Risk, A., Sear, A., Dawson, L. and Wiele, R. (1978) Midwifery, 1977. *American Journal of Obstetrics and Gynecology, 130* (8), 917–26.

Fisher, C. (1981) Community midwife: The gentle approach. *Nursing Focus, 3* (4), 562.

Flint, C. (1982) Antenatal clinics. *Nursing Mirror* (24 November; 1st, 8th, 15th and 22nd December; 5th, 12th, 19th and 26th January 1983), *155* (21–24); *156* (1–4).

Flint, C. and Poulengeris, P. (1987) *The "Know Your Midwife" Report.* Published by C. Flint, 49 Peckarmans Wood, Sydenham Hill, London.

Garcia, J. (1982) Women's views of antenatal care. In Enkin, M. and Chalmers, I. (eds), *Effectiveness and satisfaction in antenatal care.* Spastics International Medical Publications, William Heinemann Medical Books, Ltd, London.

Garcia, J., Garforth, S. and Ayers, S. (1985) Midwives confined? Labour ward policies and routines in *Research and the Midwife Conference Proceedings, 1985.* Nursing Research Unit, King's College, University of London, London.

Gilligan, M. (1980) The midwife's contribution to counselling parents who have suffered a perinatal death. *Research and the Midwife Conference Proceedings 1979* and *1980.* Chelsea College, London University, London.

Goodley, S. (1986) Family care and the preterm baby. *Midwives Chronicle, 99,* (1176), Initiatives in Care Supplement, viii–x.

Grant, A. (1984) Foreword in *Perinatal Nursing.* P.A. Field, (ed.) Churchill Livingstone, Edinburgh.

Henderson, C. (1984) Influences and interactions surrounding the midwife's decision to rupture the membranes, in *Research and the Midwife Conference Proceedings, 1984.* Nursing Research Unit, King's College, London University, London.

Hughes, P. (1986) Neonatal Community Liaison Visiting. *Midwives Chronicle, 99* (1176), Supplement, xi–xii.

Humphrey, C. (1985) The Community Midwife in Maternity Care. *Midwife Health Visitor and Community Nurse, 21* (10), 349–55.

International Congress of Midwives/International Federation of Gynaecology and Obstetrics (1973) *Definitions of the Midwife.* ICM Notices 1973.

Levy, B., Wilkinson, E. and Marine, W. (1971) Reducing neonatal mortality rate with nurse-midwives. *American Journal of Obstetrics and Gynecology, 109* (1), 50–58.

London Health Care Planning Consortium (1981) *Primary health care in Inner London* (the Acheson report), London Health Care Planning Consortium.

Maclean, G.D. (1980) Where have all the midwives gone? *Midwives Chronicle, 93* (1108), 158.

Maternity Services Advisory Committee (1982) *Maternity care in action, Part I: Antenatal care.* HMSO, London.

Morgan, B.M., Bulpitt, C.J., Clifton, P. and Lewis, P.J. (1984) The consumer attitude to obstetric care. *British Journal of Obstetrics and Gynaecology, 90* (1), 624–28.

Morrin, H.A. (1982) Are we in danger of extinction? *Midwives Chronicle, 95* (1128), 17.

Mulkerrins, M. and Gunn, P. (1985) The midwives' participation in a confidential enquiry into perinatal death conducted by the North West Thames Regional Health Authority, in *Research and the Midwife Conference Proceedings, 1985.* Nursing Research Unit, King's College, London University, London.

National Childbirth Trust (1981) *Change in antenatal care.* Report of a working party set up for the NCT by Sheila Kitzinger. National Childbirth Trust, London.

Newson, K. (1985) Breaking away from routine care. *Nursing Mirror, 161* (3), Midwifery Supplement, 18–21.

Oakley, A. (1976) Wise woman and medicine man. In Mitchell, J. and Oakley, A. (eds), *The rights and wrongs of women,* Penguin, Harmondsworth.

Oakley, A. (1984) *The Captured Womb. A History of the Medical Care of Pregnant Women.* Basil Blackwell, Oxford.

Oakley, A. and Elbourne, D. (in press) Interventions to alleviate stress in pregnancy. In Enkin, M., Keirse, M. and Chalmers, I. (eds), *Effective care in pregnancy and childbirth,* Oxford University Press, Oxford.

Penny, Y. (1986) Modern prenatal management: Pattern of care for the future. *Midwives Chronicle, 99* (1126), Supplement, ii–iii.

Raisler, J. (1985) Improving pregnancy outcome with nurse-midwifery care. *Journal of Nurse-Midwifery, 30* (4), 189–91.

Rider, A. (1983) Report on Dettol Sword Award. *Midwives Chronicle, 96* (1444), 165.

Robinson, S. (1980) Are there enough midwives? *Nursing Times, 76* (17), 726–30.

Robinson, S. (1980) Midwifery manpower in Social Services Committee on perinatal and neonatal mortality, Vol. V. HMSO, London.

Robinson, S., Golden, J. and Bradley, S. (1983) *A study of the role and responsibilities of the midwife.* NERU Report no. 1, Nursing Education Research Unit, King's College London University.

Robinson, S. (1985a) Normal maternity care: Whose responsibility? *British Journal of Obstetrics and Gynaecology, 92* (1), 1–3.

Robinson, S. (1985b) Responsibilities of midwives and medical staff: Findings from a national survey. *Midwives Chronicle, 98* (1166), 64–71.

Robinson, S. (1985c) Midwives, obstetricians and general practitioners: The need for role clarification. *Midwifery, 1* (2), 102–13.

Robinson, S. (1985d) Maternity care: A duplication of resources. *Journal of the Royal College of General Practitioners, 35.* 346–47.

Robinson, S. (1985e) Providing maternity care in the community: Some aspects of the role of the midwife, Part I. *Midwife, Health Visitor and Community Nurse, 21* (7), 222–28.

Robinson, S. (1985f) Providing maternity care in the community: Some aspects of the role of the midwife, Part 2. *Midwife, Health Visitor and Commmunity Nurse, 21* (8) 274–79.

Roch, S. (1983) Is the midwife accountable? *Nursing Times, 79* (39), 38–9.

Roch, S. (1984) Lessons from midwifery. *Senior Nurse, 1* (21), 16–17.

Royal College of Midwives and Health Visitors Association (1982). Joint statement on antenatal preparation.

Royal College of Midwives (1977) Evidence to the Royal Commission on the National Health Service. Royal College of Midwives, London.

Royal College of Midwives (1987) *The role and education of the future midwife in the United Kingdom.* Royal College of Midwives, London.

Royal College of Obstetricians and Gynaecologists/Royal College of General Practitioners (1981) Report on training for obstetrics and gynaecology for general practitioners. Joint Working Party of the RCOG and RCGP, London.

Royal College of Obstetricians and Gynaecologists (1982) Report of the RCOG Working Party on antenatal and intrapartum care. Royal College of Obstetricians and Gynaecologists, London.

Runnerstrom, L. (1969) The effectiveness of nurse-midwifery in a supervised hospital environment. *Bulletin of the American College of Nurse Midwives,* *14* (2), 40–52.

Social Services Committee – House of Commons (1980) Report on perinatal and neonatal mortality. HMSO, London.

Slome, C., Wetherbee, H., Daly, M., Christensen, K., Meglen, H. and Thiede, H. (1976) Effectiveness of certified nurse-midwives: A prospective evaluation study. *American Journal of Obstetrics and Gynecology, 124* (2), 177–82.

Stuart, B. and Judge, E. (1984) The return of the midwife? *Midwives Chronicle, 97* (1152), 8–9.

Thompson, J.B. (1986) Safety and effectiveness of nurse midwifery care: Research review. In Rooks, H.P. and Haas, J.E. (eds), *Nurse-midwifery in America.* A report of the American College of Nurse Midwives Foundation. Washington.

Towler, J. (1981) Out of the ordinary: Park Hospital Maternity Unit. *Nursing Mirror, 152* (11), 32–3.

Towler, J. (1982) A dying species: survival and revival are up to us. *Midwives Chronicle, 95* (1136), 324–8.

Towler, J. and Brammall, J. (1986) *The midwife in history and society.* Croom Helm, Kent.

William, S., Hepburn, J. and McIlwaine, G. (1985) Consumer view of epidural analgesia. *Midwifery, 1* (1), 32–36.

World Health Organisation (1966) *The midwife in maternity care.* Technical Report Series No 331, chapter 3, Geneva.

World Health Organisation (1985) *Having a baby in Europe.* Public Health in Europe 26. World Health Organisation, Regional Office for Europe, Copenhagen.

CHAPTER THREE

Recording an obstetric history or relating to a pregnant woman? A study of the antenatal booking interview

Rosemary Methven

The aim of the research described in this chapter was to investigate whether the use of the nursing process can provide childbearing women with a better quality of care than that provided by the approach usually practised by midwives. The study was undertaken in part fulfilment of the requirements of an MSc. course at the University of Manchester and was funded by a Department of Health and Social Security Research Studentship. This meant that time and resources were not available to consider all aspects of the nursing process in relation to midwifery. It was decided therefore to focus only on assessment (the first stage of the nursing process) in the context of just one aspect of a woman's care in pregnancy: the all-important antenatal booking interview. This interview is important for two main reasons. First, it should enable the midwife to obtain a picture of the whole woman and to make baseline observations on which to plan future care and assess subsequent progress. Secondly, it is the 'shopfront' of the hospital maternity services in that it is the childbearing woman's first contact with that service. By interviewing women using a nursing process approach to their care, it was possible to evaluate the extent to which the traditional history-taking interview effectively obtained information relevant to the provision of midwifery care.

THE NURSING PROCESS AND NURSING MODELS

The nursing process is a method of giving systematic, personalized care to individual patients or clients. It is based on problem-solving theory (Dewey, 1910) and usually consists of four phases:

1. assessment (history-taking) in order to identify any personal, social, emotional, or physical health-related needs of the patient
2. planning care in a logical, systematic way in order to meet specific

goals related to the identified patient needs
3. implementation of the planned care in association with the patient and his/her relatives and other members of the health care team where appropriate
4. evaluation of the effectiveness of care given

In itself, the nursing process provides only a logical way of organizing care. It is a meaningless practice without an explicit framework or model around which the assessment and planning of care can be arranged. Each nursing model highlights particular beliefs and values held about nursing practice, that is, the patient or client, the goals and outcomes of care and the knowledge needed to achieve them. In this way, nursing models afford 'a unifying framework for an organised way of looking at nursing' (Pearson and Vaughan, 1986) and provide a pattern that gives direction and guidance to those using the nursing process.

As yet there is no model specifically designed for midwifery practice. The model used in this research was developed by Orem (1980) and was chosen because it provides for individuals to meet their own self-care needs in order to maintain personal health. The nursing role within this model is described as that of teaching, providing physical, psychological or social support, guiding, creating an environment that promotes the personal development of the client, and, where necessary, 'acting or doing for them' when they are unable to care for themselves. This philosophy was felt to be particularly appropriate to pregnancy, viewed as 'a normal, if altered state of health', and to incorporate most aspects of the role of the midwife during pregnancy, labour and the postnatal period, without reducing the women to the category of 'patient'.

Fundamental to the concept of the nursing process is the contention that a person is a holistic being with physical, psychological, social and spiritual attributes (Smutts, 1926). Also essential to the successful operation of nursing process in a ward-based setting in patient allocation rather than task allocation. Continuity of care can be achieved by following the woman's care-plan, based on a nursing process assessment, from booking right through to the end of the postnatal period, even though several different midwives may be involved in providing that care. In this way confusion and conflicting advice can be minimized (Thomson, 1980; Ball, 1981).

THE NURSING PROCESS AND MIDWIFERY: PROGRESS TO DATE

The nursing process was first introduced in midwifery in the late 1970s, with schemes set up at Stepping Hill Maternity Hospital in Stockport (Bryans, 1985), Queen Charlotte's Maternity Hospital in London (Adams *et al.*, 1981; Bryar 1986) and in two other London maternity hospitals (Whitfield, 1983). These pioneering efforts were initiated when 'there was no reference to the use of nursing process in midwifery in Britain' (Adams *et al.*, 1981). Bryar (1987) notes that 'a computer search in 1981 yielded only five American references to the use of nursing process in midwifery in contrast to the two hundred and forty items listed in the Royal College of Nursing bibliography' on the use of the nursing process in nursing. Bryar suggests that this dearth of literature indicates that midwives showed very little interest in the application of the nursing process to midwifery at that time. Bowers, Charles and Wood (1987) surveyed the views of maternity staff in relation to the use of the nursing process and concluded that its effectiveness would depend on staff attitudes and the knowledge and support of managers.

Further progress was made, however, by those convinced of its value and committed to its underlying theory and principles. Fender (1981) described the use by community midwives of the nursing process, while Methven (1986b) and Keane (1982) demonstrated its application to the care of individual women in hospital. Gibbs (1983) explained the adaptation of the nursing process to meet the needs of patients on a neonatal unit, and Ball and Stanley (1984) showed that in the postnatal ward a care plan increased discussion of individual needs, reduced the use of routinized care in favour of more individually planned care, and increased midwives' responsibility for decision-making. These findings are borne out by the Stockport experience, where improved staff morale, reduced sickness and absence rates, and less paperwork were reported as the outcomes of introducing the nursing process into the maternity hospital (Bryans, 1985).

A number of authors discuss the need for the nursing process in relation to improved record-keeping and documentation of the woman's needs in childbirth (Thomson, 1980; Flint, 1983; Methven, 1986a). In some areas, consumers of the midwifery services have also shown considerable interest in the potential of nursing process documentation in allowing individual choice in the management of labour (Kitzinger, 1983).

Whitfield (1983) admits that progress has been slower than expected, but five years after her original statement, Bryar (1987) concludes that British midwives are now beginning to show some interest in the nursing process and to apply it in practice. The inclusion of the nursing process within the English National Board (ENB) syllabus for midwifery training should go some way to accelerating this, provided that those responsible for teaching and implementing nursing process in midwifery are themselves thoroughly conversant with its principles and practice. In 1986 the ENB Learning Resources Unit published a guide book on the 'planned, individualised care of mother, baby and the family unit' (Heath *et al.*, 1986).

METHODS

Research design

The study had two phases: the traditional booking interview and the antenatal interview using a nursing process assessment format.

Phase 1: The traditional booking interview. As described below, phase 1 had three stages.

Stage 1: Description of the booking interview. A descriptive study of the booking interview was undertaken in order to determine the content and quality of the information recorded about the woman in her obstetric notes and the process by which the midwife obtained this information. The conversation between the mother and the midwife was tape-recorded. However, as Birdwhistell (1968) observed, only 35% of communication is transmitted verbally and so the researcher observed and recorded on a checklist the non-verbal aspects of the interaction. These included posture, facial expression, eye behaviour, bodily movement, overall manner and vocal para-language (e.g. laughter, sighs and grunts) made by the midwife and the woman. The use of a stopwatch and time scale made it possible to add these features to the transcribed recording of their verbal conversation, thus providing a script of both verbal and non-verbal exchange between interviewer and interviewee.

The content of the booking interview, both verbal and non-verbal, was compared with a list of criteria considered to constitute an ideal antenatal booking interview. This list was developed by reference to several textbooks of midwifery and obstetric practice (Bailey, 1972; Browne and Dixon, 1978; Myles, 1981; Towler and Butler-Manuel, 1980). Colleagues working in antenatal clinics and midwifery teaching departments were also approached with a request for criteria for the ideal booking interview, against which those being developed as a research tool could be validated. It was decided that the list of criteria should include those in the current conventional booking interview as indicated on the antenatal front sheet (the first page of the mother's obstetric record on the medical notes), and those features that could be expected in a nursing process assessment. The list included the following: general data on address, marital status, occupation and religion, general medical history, obstetric history, history of present pregnancy (physical and social) and pattern of antenatal care.

Stage 2: Midwives' views of the antenatal booking interview. Using a semi-structured schedule, the researcher interviewed the interviewing midwife about various aspects of the antenatal booking interview. These included the midwife's views of the adequacy of her own preparation for interviewing women during pregnancy, and her views on additional education midwives require in this respect. She was also asked for her views on the role of medical staff in the booking interview and the role that the nursing process might have in midwifery care. The full list of questions is shown in Appendix A.

Stage 3: Women's views of the antenatal booking interview. Each of the women was asked to complete a questionnaire covering various aspects of her experience of the interview (see Appendix B).

Phase 2: Antenatal interview using a nursing process assessment formula. The researcher then carried out a semi-structured interview with the woman using a nursing process assessment format based on the self-care model of Orem (1980). Content criteria of the nursing process assessment came from relevant literature (McCain, 1965; Marriner, 1969; Robinson, 1978; Orem, 1980); the assessment is included as Appendix C. It was important that this exercise did not reduce the credibility of the interviewing midwife or the hospital's system of care in the eyes of the mother. For this reason, a deliberate decision was taken not to duplicate areas of enquiry already covered by the booking interview.

The overall research design for Phase 1 is illustrated in Fig. 3.1.

The design made it possible to compare the traditional history-taking interview with a nursing process-style assessment in order to gauge the degree to which each resulted in information on which the woman's midwifery care could be based. It also went some way to answering the initial research question: Can the nursing process provide a better quality of care for women and their babies than the approach habitually practised by midwives?

The sample. Constraints of time and money meant that a maximum of 40 antenatal booking interviews could be observed. Ten women from

Figure 3.1 The research design for Phase 1.

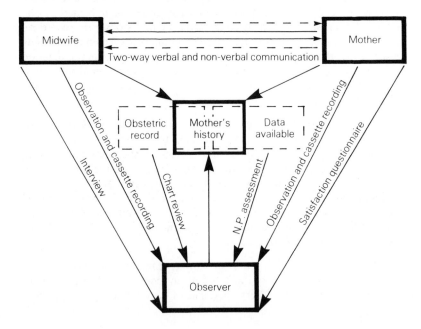

each of four hospitals were selected in order to avoid a possible bias that might have resulted from studying the practices in one unit only. The four hospitals were chosen to represent a range of size, location and practice, and included a purpose-built maternity hospital serving a modern housing estate, an older teaching hospital within the inner city, a maternity unit within a large teaching hospital with a multiracial catchment area and a small maternity unit forming part of a district general hospital complex on the edge of the city serving an urban and rural population. All hospitals were approved as training institutions for student midwives.

The women were to be approached personally as they registered at the clinic and asked to participate in the study. The only subjects excluded from the study were those unable to speak English and those who were accompanied to the clinic by a partner or friend. The latter were excluded as participation in the study would have meant separation for most of the three-hour booking visit, which was felt to be unacceptable. Forty-three women were asked to participate, of whom three declined.

Gaining access. Permission for the study was obtained from the relevant staff in each hospital, an enlightening experience that provided insight into the way these groups of staff viewed research. In hospital A, permission was granted even before the details of the study had been outlined to the Divisional Nursing Officer. However, her counterpart at hospital B was concerned about the questionnaire to be completed by the mother but untroubled by the recording of the booking interview because, 'it's what they do all the time'. Therefore, it was necessary to request permission from the ethical committee, who considered the abstract of the research proposal. They felt the sample size was too small to be meaningful and expressed doubts about the relevance of the study. The chairman, an obstetrician who only practised gynaecology, commented: 'The midwife plays such an insignificant part in the overall initial visit to clinic by mothers at this hospital, that I wonder if it is worthwhile doing a study on such a small part'. Eventually, with the approval of the rest of the committee, the chairman agreed the study could take place although, in his view, it was 'a waste of time'.

At the smallest hospital (C), it was necessary to be present at the weekly obstetric meeting attended by all medical staff, from consultant to medical students. There was a fairly heated discussion about the questions to be asked, question phrasing, questionnaire design and inter-view technique. Various hypothetical situations were then posed in order to test the reaction and response that might be forthcoming if anything similar were to be encountered in reality. They felt 'computerized obstet-ric records' were the obvious solution as the midwife 'only had about five minutes with each mother and no opportunity to form a relationship with her'. Permission was finally granted. In the final hospital (D), the Senior Nursing Officer obtained permission for access on behalf of the researcher from the senior obstetrician.

Staff working in the antenatal clinics each received a letter explaining how the study was to be conducted and asking for their willingness to participate. They were not told the purpose of the study in detail in an attempt to reduce a possible 'Hawthorne' effect (Roesthlisberger and Dickson, 1939). They were told that the study would 'help midwives to know whether any changes are needed in the present system of antenatal care and to assist mothers in future to receive the type of care they prefer'. Two midwives who did not wish to be observed and recorded opted out of the study. Twenty-eight midwives participated, including the four midwives in charge of each of the antenatal clinics. Some were observed more than once.

Preliminary testing of strategy. Before undertaking the pilot study, it was essential to ensure that aspects of the interview being assessed were similar in each hospital. This preliminary investigation made it possible to assess when and where the midwife could be interviewed and the woman could complete the satisfaction questionnaire without losing her place in the queue or lengthening the overall time spent in the clinic. The researcher achieved this by accompanying two women from each hospital in the study from the moment they entered the clinic, through each stage of their booking visit until they left the building. This exercise confirmed the feasibility and logistics of carrying out the study.

The pilot study. The pilot study demonstrated how long it took to select a woman, secure her willingness to participate in the study, record the interview, administer the questionnaire, and conduct the nursing process interview. Minor adjustments were made to the checklist, interview schedule and questionnaire.

DATA COLLECTION AND ANALYSIS

The data collected consisted of:

- 40 cassette recordings of the booking interview which were transcribed by the researcher for subsequent analysis
- 40 observation sheets which were correlated with the interview transcripts
- 40 post-booking interview questionnaires completed by the women
- 28 summaries of interviews with midwives in change of clinics and those who had been observed taking one or more histories from women
- 40 copies of data recorded on the antenatal front sheet of the women's obstetric record
- 40 nursing process assessment interviews

Each hospital had its own format for the antenatal front sheet but the material to be recorded on each one covered similar subject areas: personal information; social data; medical, surgical and family history;

obstetric record and history of present pregnancy. However, some hospitals were more explicit in the information required. For example, hospital A asked for 'pregnancy complications', which prompted the interviewing midwives to probe specifically about any admission during pregnancy, raised blood pressure, or urinary tract infection. Hospital B's heading was merely 'antenatal' which encouraged the interviewing midwife to ask 'Was everything all right in pregnancy?' or 'Did you have a normal pregnancy?' These differences contributed to the way questions were asked and consequently to the quality and quantity of information obtained from the woman.

The main aspects of data collection and analysis for each stage of the research are described below.

Analysis of the content and process of the antenatal booking interview

Content. The interview content was assessed by completing a criteria checklist and comparing this with the previously compiled list of criteria for the ideal booking interview.

The results indicated only that the topics were discussed during the interview and are not a measure of the quality of the interaction that occurred or of the information sought. It would require another, more sensitive tool to investigate the quality of the items included, and whether the questions did constitute 'effective probing'.

Process. Measurement of the interview process was more complicated. At the time this study was undertaken, existing work on communication in nursing had concentrated on aspects of normal conversation. As these interviews consisted of question-and-answer type responses, no existing tool for analysis could be found. Thus, one was developed using de Julia's (1980) nursing interview for classifying interview style, the Open University's list of interviewing skills (1979), and Maguire and Rutter's (1976) model developed for medical students for classifying interview technique. The resulting categories used for analysis are shown in Table 3.1.

The interactive skills used by the midwives during the booking interview were analysed first and then the transcripts were analysed again to identify the interview techniques employed. The guidelines for interview skills listed by the Open University (1979), as shown below, were used for analysing the booking interview interaction. These included:

1. putting the respondent at ease
2. asking questions in an interested manner
3. noting the responses without interrupting the conversation
4. giving support without introducing bias
5. drawing the interaction to a satisfactory conclusion.

A further category, entitled 'Interview Opportunity', was added; this

Table 3.1 Final categories used for classification of midwives' interviewing skills

---

Interactive Style

1. Closed questions

    dichotomous question
    forced or fixed alternative
    multiple question
    negative question
    contracted question

2. Direct questions

3. Leading questions

    persuasive question
    biased question
    partly-answered question
    unfinished question
    validatory question

4. Non-Directive questions

    general question
    rhetorical question

5. Open questions

Interview Technique

1. Developing devices

    prompting
    probing

2. Facilitating devices

    verbal facilitation
    non-verbal facilitation
    mirroring or reflection
    unintended facilitation

3. Controlling devices

    verification
    changing the conversation
    transfer
    use of cliches

4. Other reactions

    empathy
    approval or disapproval
    laughter
    perception of non-verbal cues
    lateral/vertical communication
    formal/informal communication

Interview Opportunity

1. Giving information or advice

2. Explanation

3. Instruction

4. Education

Source: Compiled by the author.

was an analysis of the extent to which the interviewing midwife used the opportunity of the antenatal booking interview for giving information, advice, explanation, instruction or education to the mother as well as recording the information obtained from her.

Analysis of the assessment interview based on Orem's (1980) self-care model

The responses of each mother were categorized under headings related to the eight universal health care requisites defined by Orem's model as shown below. Figures in brackets refer to the questions on the interview schedule that relate to this particular health care requisite (Appendix C).

1. the maintenance of a sufficient intake of food (1a–1g)
2. the maintenance of a sufficient intake of water (2a–2e)
3. the provision of care associated with elimination processes and excrements (5a–5i)
4. the maintenance of a sufficient intake of air (4a–4b)
5. the maintenance of a balance between activity and rest (3a–3g)
6. the prevention of hazard to human life, human functioning and human well-being (8a–8h)
7. the maintenance of a balance between solitude and social interaction (9a–9i)
8. promotion of human functioning and development with social groups in accord with human potential, known human limitations and the human desire to be normal (6a–6i)

As well as summarizing the data obtained from the total sample of 40 mothers, findings for one mother, selected at random, were examined in detail. The data from her assessment interview was compared to that obtained by the midwife at the antenatal booking interview and recorded on the front sheet of the mother's obstetric record. Immediately the difference in the effectiveness of each interview method in gathering data relevant for midwifery care was apparent. From the assessment data, needs expressed by the mother and problems identified by the researcher were then organized so that a nursing process care plan could be designed. Goals of care were identified and a hypothetical plan of care to meet these goals was devised; this has been reported elsewhere (Methven, 1986a).

FINDINGS

Conduct and content of the antenatal booking interview

The findings from this phase of the research are presented under the following headings: midwives' interviewing skills, the relationship between the content of the interview and the criteria checklist, the midwifery and/or obstetric orientation of the interview, the written record of the interview, and the relationship formed between the midwife and the woman.

Interviewing skills employed by midwives. By far the majority of questions used by all midwives in every interview were closed in structure. In most instances, use of the closed question was appropriate because the interviewers were seeking specific, factual answers. To be effective, however, the closed question needs to be correctly worded and accurately phrased. The following example shows how the midwife received an answer to the question asked. If she had not rephrased the question, inaccurate information could have been recorded.

Midwife: OK, so this is your second baby?
Woman (quietly): Yes.
Midwife: Have you ever had any miscarriages or terminations or any other pregnancies that haven't gone ...?
Woman: Er ... yes. I did have a termination when I was 20.
Midwife: So you have been pregnant three times, including this one?
Woman: Yes.

By use of the closed question, the midwife effectively controlled the interview. Several instances were recorded in which erroneous data were written on the notes either because a closed question was not structured correctly or because the mother was not given an opportunity to qualify her answer.

There was abundant evidence in the 40 interviews to support the conclusion of MacLeod Clark (1981) that 'consistent, or habitual use of closed questions produces a powerful influence which will control or block development of a conversation'. Every interview in the study contained a sequence similar to this. As the interaction developed, the pace increased and the tone of both mother and midwife rose correspondingly.

Midwife: Have you had any previous pregnancies at all?
Woman: No.
Midwife: Have you had any blood transfusions?
Woman: No.
Midwife: Have you had any operations at all?
Woman: No.
Midwife: Have you had any illnesses like TB?
Woman: No.
Midwife: Rheumatic fever?
Woman: No.
Midwife: Diabetes?
Woman: No.
Midwife: Heart problems?
Woman: No.

and so on.

The second largest group of questions to be used was the 'leading question', which suggested or encouraged the respondent to reply in a certain way. This is generally considered to be a bad technique as it influences the information that is recorded about the mother. The most frequently found example was: 'You are going to breastfeed your baby, aren't you?' Such encouragement no doubt stems from the *Midwife's Code of Practice* (Central Midwives Board, 1978), which directed the midwife to 'promote breast feeding'.

Non-directive questions have been defined by de Julia (1980) as those that are 'general in nature and can be answered in a variety of ways. They are used to encourage the patient to talk'. Such questions were noticeable by their absence. When asked, they were frequently followed by a direct question before the mother had time to reply, thus negating the effect of the original enquiry.

Only three open questions were identified in the 40 interviews. According to de Julia (1980), 'open questions are those which allow the patient to express freely what he thinks and feels'. Pressure of time may have prevented more of these questions being asked, or it could have been that the obstetric notes did not provide space for this type of information to be recorded. It is also possible that the interviewing midwives were not interested in obtaining this sort of information about women, and did not view them holistically but rather as obstetric objects.

Interview technique, assessed against the criteria set out in the model for interviewing developed by Maguire and Rutter (1976), indicated that midwives demonstrated very few devices for developing conversation or for probing in order to obtain salient facts. It is suggested that the style of questioning and interview technique were influenced primarily by pressure of time and workload, and secondly by poor role models when skills were being learnt. In addition, the Central Midwives Board syllabus for midwifery training prescribed very little, if any, specific teaching about actual interviewing skills in either classroom or clinical situations at that time.

Relationship between content of the observed booking interview and the criteria checklist

Very few of the checklist topics were covered at every interview in the study. This is illustrated in Table 3.2 which shows a section of the checklist and the number of times each of the criteria was raised. The highest scores were for the woman's family history, closely followed by her personal history and smoking habits; these items are clearly indicated on the antenatal front sheet of the woman's obstetric records. The midwives revealed in their personal interviews that they used the front sheets as an interview checklist. Tables 3.3 and 3.4 illustrate the variety of topics specified on the antenatal front sheet in each hospital. It would be interesting to know if women who were asked if they had ever had a 'squint', for example, received care that was in any way different from

Table 3.2 Section of content of antenatal booking interview

History of present pregnancy	Hospital*			
	A	B	C	D
1. Menstrual History				
Probing questions used effectively to establish:				
First day of last normal period	10	9	9	10
Her certainty *re* the date	3	8	7	10
Normality of period in duration	3		2	2
amount	2	1	2	2
Any further bleeding since, date/gestation (where appropriate)	1	9	2	9
Its nature			2	2
Its amount		1	2	2
Use of oral contraceptive prior to pregnancy	9	10	10	8
Date oral contraception discontinued	6	5	9	5
Mother's usual menstrual cycle Frequency	10	10	8	10
Duration	9	10	8	9
Regularity	9	10	8	10
E.D.D. calculated correctly	7	4	8	3
E.D.D. validated with mother	8	6	4	9
Pregnancy test result		1	9	1
2. Mother's Pattern of Normal Living				
Appropriate probing questions used to ascertain:				
State of mother's general health in pregnancy to date	8	3	1	4
Mother's usual diet	3	2		1
Usual fluid intake				1
Any changes necessitated by pregnancy				
Dietary specification in hospital				
Appropriate advice given *re* diet	4	1		
weight gain	2			
Any perceived weight gain or loss in pregnancy	1			
Consumption of alcohol		2	2	7
Appropriate advice given		1		2
Usual pattern of elimination by bladder				1
bowel				
Any changes noticed in pregnancy				
Appropriate advice given				1
Usual pattern of rest				
activity	1			1
Changes due to pregnancy	1			1
Suitability of clothing (brassière)				
shoes				

History of present pregnancy	Hospital*			
	A	B	C	D
Advice re posture in pregnancy given				
Views on contraceptive practice		1		
Smoking habit	10	10	10	10
Advice given	3	4	1	4
Dental health and state of gums		1		2
Advice re dental care in pregnancy given				2
Other feature, appliances/prostheses				
Sight or hearing loss			2	
Speech or language difficulty				
3. Social History				
Appropriate probing questions used to ascertain:				
Family situation, proximity of relatives			1	4
Their attitude to present pregnancy			1	2
Arrangements for care				
of dependants during clinic				
hospital admission				
Support available on return home			3	1
Length of time married	2		2	2
Social worker in contact	2		1	4
contact to be established	2		1	6
4. Psychological and Emotional Aspects				
Appropriate probing questions used to ascertain:				
Response to pregnancy by mother				
partner	5			2
Invited views about labour, etc	2			3
Any fears or emotions re having a baby	1			2
Views on being a mother (parent) (again)				1
Enquiry made for information not asked for			1	2

Source: Compiled by the author.
*Maximum score possible for any item is 10.

those women who were not asked that question.

The influence of the obstetric record was apparent in its effect on the order in which questions were asked. 'We start at the top and work down to the bottom,' commented one midwife. This meant that in some instances the woman's expected date of delivery was calculated from the first day of her last menstrual period and recorded on the notes. Several minutes later, when the midwife had worked down the page and asked

Table 3.3 Topics specified on the antenatal front sheet of each hospital in the study concerning the mother's personal and family medical history

	Hospital			
	A	B	C	D
Alcohol				*
Allergic disease		*		
Asthma				*
Blood transfusion	*	*	*	*
Chickenpox			*	
Congenital abnormality	*	*	*	*
Deep vein thrombosis				*
Diabetes	*	*	*	*
Dystrophies		*		
Epilepsy			*	
German measles			*	
Heart disease				*
Hepatitis				*
Hypertension		*	*	
Measles			*	
Medications/current drug therapy	*	*		*
Mumps			*	
Operations			*	*
Poliomyelitis			*	
Psychiatric disorders	*			
Pulmonary embolus				*
Renal disease				*
Rheumatic fever	*		*	*
Road traffic accident			*	
Sensitivities to drugs or agents	*	*	*	*
Smoking	*	*	*	*
Squint				*
Tuberculosis	*	*	*	*
Twins	*	*	*	*

Source: Compiled by the author.

about the woman's use of contraceptives, it became apparent that the date had sometimes been calculated from a ('pill') withdrawal bleed.

The design of the obstetric records influenced the type of question asked by the midwife. Where there was a box to be filled with a tick or short word, a closed question would be used. Where a general heading, such as 'previous pregnancy' was written, the midwife was more likely to use a non-directive question, which resulted in information of a more useful quality being obtained.

Table 3.4 Topics specified on the antenatal front sheet of each hospital in the study concerning the mother's past obstetric history

	Hospital			
	A	B	C	D
Date	*	*	*	*
Antenatal period/pregnancy	*	*		*
Gestation/maturity	*		*	*
Labour/delivery				*
duration/length	*	*		
method of delivery	*	*	*	*
Where confined	*	*	*	
Puerperium	*	*		*
Complications of Preg./Lab./Puerp.			*	
Alive/S.B./N.N.D.	*	*	*	*
Sex	*	*	*	
Weight	*	*	*	*
Feeding baby	*			
Health now		*	*	

Source: Compiled by the author.

Midwives experienced in interviewing frequently followed a general question, such as 'Was everything all right after delivery?', with more probing questions that referred to specific events. Midwives inexperienced in interviewing did not have this facility and much important information was never obtained, as the second phase of the study demonstrates.

Two women were asked if they had had any operations and both gave a negative reply. However, both had had a miscarriage. Further questioning by the interviewing midwives revealed that a cervical dilatation and uterine curretage had been undertaken following the miscarriages. Without such probing, inaccurate information would have been recorded because the women were apparently unaware that a dilatation and curretage constituted an 'operation'.

These examples serve to demonstrate that, for a variety of reasons, the content of the interviews varied in quality and quantity. In some cases, the reality of what should have been written will never be known. In others, there was clear evidence of error, or omission. It is disturbing to note that the record on which the woman's subsequent care is based may contain erroneous or inadequate information.

Midwifery/Obstetric orientation of the interview. The influence of the design of the front sheet of the obstetric notes has already been mentioned. It was also apparent that topics not specifically mentioned on the front sheet tended not to be asked (see Tables 3.3 and 3.4 and Appendix C). The result in terms of the content of the interview was a substantial amount of data concerning medical and obstetric history, but practically nothing about the woman's responses to child-birth, her feelings concerning her present pregnancy, and her views on the management of her past or present confinement.

Midwives did not avail themselves of the opportunity to ask about breast feeding apart from ascertaining by which method the next baby was to be fed. One woman who had tried desperately to breast feed her first child without success, tried repeatedly to talk to the interviewing midwife about what went wrong and how she might succeed this time. Their conversation was as follows:

> Midwife (without looking up from the notes she was writing): Have you tried shells?
> Woman: Yes, I tried everything last time. I would willingly give it another try so that it would be better, but I just think I'd be losing the battle. (Tone of voice indicated she wanted help.)
> Midwife: OK, love. (Records 'Not breast feeding, inverted nipples, has tried shells' on the woman's notes.) Fine, all done.

The midwife then marched from the room, leaving the bewildered woman to follow.

Data on interview techniques suggested that the interviews were obstetrically oriented, as, for example, with the use of the technique cate-gorized as 'transfer'. It was frequently employed, especially by junior or inexperienced midwives. Instead of accepting the responsibility to answer a question, make a decision, or give advice that had been asked for, the midwife would transfer the situation to another member of staff, usually a doctor. The following excerpt of a conversation took place during a mother's interview with an experienced staff midwife.

> Woman: The only thing that's not really worrying me, it's just on my mind, you know, with Christopher being premature ...
> Midwife: Yes, you know they'll have to sort this thing out when you see the obstetrician. He's the one that is going to look after you during pregnancy.

The midwife did not take time to discover the real nature of the woman's anxiety. She assumed that it was a problem that should be referred to an obstetrician. The woman's concern may well have been of a much more practical nature and well within the midwife's capability for advice, re-assurance, or specific help. If not, the precise problem should have been identified and then the woman referred to the most appropriate person, who might have been the obstetrician. The attitude displayed would surely discourage any woman seeking further help from a midwife in the future.

The conversation continued:

Woman: It's just that, you know, with everything going OK before, you know, with it still being premature, you know.
Midwife: The thing is, anytime, if you are worried, you know you can just phone in, they'll always ...
Woman: (breaks in) I know, they'll always say they'll, they'll ...
(The woman's frustration to make herself understood and get her point across is apparent.) You know, two pregnancies aren't the same, you know.
Midwife: They'll sort that out and —
Woman: (hollow laugh)
Midwife: — take all that into consideration, but mention it to them, that it's worrying you.
Woman: Yes.
Midwife: So they'll, they will take time to explain everything, you know.
Woman: Yes.
Midwife: Right, now where are we? June '82. (She calculates the mother's expected date of delivery and continues with the remainder of the interview according to the order prescribed by the obstetric record.)

Most of the midwives observed appeared to be inflexible in their approach to the interview, as the example above illustrates. The majority were unable to cover the material in any order other than that prescribed by the notes, and resisted attempts by the woman to ask questions that might deflect them from that set pattern.

The conclusion from these findings is that the antenatal booking interview as currently undertaken is oriented towards obstetrics rather than midwifery, conforming to a medical rather than a midwifery model. It is suggested that, in consequence, midwives are unwittingly regarding the childbearing woman as an obstetric object rather than a person with hopes and fears, views and opinions, personality and relationships within a unique social context. In addition, midwives are not availing themselves of the opportunity to establish a supportive relationship within which women feel encouraged to discuss any problems or concerns they may have.

The written record of the interview. Generally, the information about the woman was recorded neatly and legibly. However, for the majority of obstetric notes there was little opportunity for longhand, and even less for detailed explanation. Most of the facts were recorded as ticks or crosses in boxes. Possible reasons for some omissions or inaccuracies have already been suggested. Abbreviations further increased the problem, as, for example, one record read: 'Sister's brother's child has S.B.' However, the 'S.B.' in question was not a stillbirth but a child with spina bifida. The later nursing process assessment revealed that the brother-in-law had not one, but two, children with this condition.

The amount of conversation that took place that was not recorded on the notes depended a great deal on the skill of the interviewer in making the woman talk. When the front sheet was used as a questionnaire, questions were asked in a closed format and little additional information was obtained. Furthermore, if additional facts did surface, there was usually no place to write them in the notes and, in consequence, that information went unrecorded. It is possible that these limitations affected the midwives' interview style and influenced what questions they asked and how they asked them. If there was no space to record how the mother was reacting to her pregnancy, why bother to enquire? The later nursing process assessment demonstrated how much information relevant to a woman's midwifery care was available, but was never ascertained and therefore never recorded.

The relationship formed between the midwife and the woman at the booking interview. Data for this analysis were obtained from the researcher's interview with the midwives as well as the transcribed conversations between woman and midwife at booking.

Of the 28 midwives questioned, 26 were emphatic that a midwife was the best person to conduct the booking interview. Six felt that 'a woman can always relate better with a woman'. Other reasons given were that 'midwives appreciate what midwives need to know. It's separate knowledge from what the doctor needs to know. Midwives understand the implication of questions and replies and can question the woman further.' Five midwives stated that 'a bond needs to be formed between the mother and the midwife if the midwife is to care for her for the rest of her pregnancy'.

Analysis of the data revealed a clear distinction between the views of midwives who worked permanently in the antenatal clinic and those who were there for a short time as part of a rotational programme. The ten permanent midwives were emphatic that a relationship with the woman was always formed during the booking interview. 'It's automatic', said one of them. In contrast, the other group of midwives, while acknowledging that it was possible to form a relationship with the woman at booking, demonstrated techniques in their interview style that appeared to deliberately prevent this occurring. In response to further questioning about this, they revealed that their lack of permanence in the clinic affected their willingness to form a relationship with the woman; they were unsure if they would see the woman again and so deliberately tried not to get too involved with her during the interview.

It is interesting that the midwives who were most convinced that a relationship was formed during booking conducted the fewest interviews. The all-important task of establishing a relationship with the woman and obtaining the information on which her future care would be based was given to the least experienced, non-permanent clinic staff. These midwives were the very ones who were not able to take advantage of the opportunity to form a relationship with the woman and develop it on a long-term basis. Those midwives who knew best what information was most needed for a woman's care and were in a position to maintain a relationship with her throughout pregnancy, delegated this function in order that they could perform the all-important task, as they saw it, of 'keeping an eye on the doctors' and chaperoning them while the mother was being examined.

In contrast, the women's views on the relationship formed with the interviewing midwife fell into three groups. Fifteen felt that a relationship had been formed with her, another fifteen felt just as strongly that a relationship had not been formed with her, while the remaining ten women were undecided.

Analysis of the midwife's interview technique revealed little evidence of any deliberate attempt to develop a rapport or form a relationship with the woman. Ten interviews contained a long introductory explanation by the midwife that was interpreted as an attempt to put the mother at ease and so pave the way for an effective rapport and subsequent relationship; six of these took place in the same hospital. Twenty-five interviews began with no more introduction than: 'Right, first of all, I'd like to ask you a few things about yourself, your history, your medical history, and then about your family conditions. OK? Have you ever suffered from diabetes? . . .' Eleven interviews had even less introduction than this.

Five interviews were felt to demonstrate a real attempt by the midwife to establish a relationship with the woman before commencing factual questioning. This was achieved by asking interested questions about the mother's background, journey to clinic, and home circumstances at the same time as the personal data, already recorded and typed onto the case notes, were being validated.

It is significant that the only three midwives to address the woman by name during the interview were all placed in the 'validation' category of introduction. Only one midwife introduced herself by name and grade to the woman, which may help to explain why 51% of mothers were unable to identify the interviewer as a midwife. Even more disturbing was the midwives' failure to use the mother's name. Twenty-three women were never referred to by their name once they had been called for interview. Another 14 were addressed impersonally by their surname in order to check that the notes corresponded to the person being interviewed.

Data on the manner in which a midwife drew the interview to a conclusion demonstrated the lack of relationship formation. In 33 interviews, the midwife terminated the interaction by ushering the woman on to the next phase of her booking clinic visit. It was the most impersonal aspect of a largely impersonal interview and confirmed the comments of those midwives who stated that they did not want to develop a relationship in case they did not meet the woman again. Typical remarks were 'I'll leave you here to go and see the doctor' or 'I'll show you where to go.' Fifteen women were asked if they had any questions, although for one midwife, this was obviously an afterthought as she escorted the woman through the door. Only one midwife indicated a future meeting when the woman returned for her next appointment. Two said 'bye bye' as they parted, and six assured the woman that she could contact the hospital by telephone if she had any queries before her next appointment.

Four interviews were classed as 'dismissal' because the midwife finished her questions and simply left the woman without a word of explanation or farewell. There was no mechanism for the woman and midwife to meet again during the booking visit. Two women, after a pause, asked the researcher in a bemused sort of way, 'What happens now?' One was collected by another sister and escorted to wait for the doctor. The other woman, having experience from a previous pregnancy, gathered up her things and returned to the waiting area. Another interview in this category has been described above (see page 52).

The way in which the interviews were concluded demonstrated that generally the interaction was impersonal, ritualized, and mostly undertaken with what Clark (1978) has described as the attitude of 'getting through the work'.

Findings from the nursing process assessment based on Orem (1980)

The first question of the nursing process assessment related to the woman's ability to eat sufficient amounts of the right kind of food. Midwives have always been taught that a well-balanced diet of 2500 calories per day is recommended in pregnancy (Myles, 1981). This should be fairly evenly distributed between three meals each day. Of the 40 mothers questioned about their lunch:

    16 ate a sandwich
    11 had a light snack
     5 ate nothing
     1 had a pack of crisps
     1 had a pint of milk and an orange
     1 had a cup of soup and a yoghurt

Further questioning revealed that the women who appeared to be on a diet lunch did not eat anything substantial at any other point in the day, so that their overall nutritional intake was grossly inadequate, especially considering they were pregnant. The majority of mothers had 'a bowl of cereal' for breakfast and five had a regular evening meal of 'biscuits and cheese'.

Two of the women who were judged to have an inadequate diet also came into the 'heavy drinker' category, that is, they drank five or more units of alcohol per day (Plant, 1986). When questioned about her urinary output, one of these women replied, 'I only ever go once a day', while the other one said, 'I go all day without going, I only go once a day, about five o'clock.' It was this woman who stated that she ate 'seven packets of crisps each day' and not much else. It was felt that both these women need a great deal of information about diet and health and possibly some medical supervision as well. Unfortunately, their obstetric records provided no indication of their state of health or lifestyle.

The question 'How did you feel when you first realized that you were pregnant?' yielded three distinct classes of reaction. Everyone answered spontaneously and decisively in a single word or short staccato sentences. Eighteen of the women were definitely pleased to be pregnant, replying 'overjoyed', 'thrilled', or 'great'. Nine women expressed some mixed feeling and were 'uncertain if it was true' or 'couldn't believe it'. The remainding 13 women were shocked to discover they were pregnant and made statements such as 'I felt really scared', 'horrified', 'shattered', or 'petrified'.

By the time that some of these women came to the booking clinic, their initial responses to the pregnancy had changed. Only 15 women were pleased about being pregnant, but now 17 had mixed feelings and only eight were definitely 'not happy'. Some women had become aware of the responsibility of parenthood or were facing up to the financial implications of having a baby. Several women who had had a previous miscarriage relaxed once the first 12 weeks had passed and so entered the 'pleased' group. In contrast to the information obtained from the conventional booking history, these women readily came across as individuals. It is suggested that this is a very revealing way of discovering whether a pregnancy is a wanted or planned affair without having to ask intrusive, direct questions that may cause embarrassment to both the woman and midwife. It is also felt that with the knowledge of a woman's feelings about her pregnancy, the midwife is able to respond appropriately and share the woman's joy and excitement or assist her to come to terms with an unwanted situation.

The major significance of this style of interviewing was apparent when the data recorded about the woman was compared with that recorded in her antenatal notes. The nursing process assessment interview provided a mass of pertinent, factual detail relevant to a woman's midwifery and sometimes her obstetric care. But in every case she emerged as a person in her own right, with views and feelings about her baby, opinions about her care and management in pregnancy and labour. Her family, activities of daily living and her present physiological and psychological responses to pregnancy were also brought into focus. The data on one woman were further analysed to make a hypothetical care plan (Methven, 1986), from which a nursing process system of care could have been given. Time did not allow such an analysis to be made of each woman in the study, but this would certainly be possible. In summary, the comparison of the content of the traditional antenatal booking history with the nursing process assessment interview revealed that the former was woefully inadequate both in quality and quantity.

CONCLUSIONS AND RECOMMENDATIONS

The majority of interviews observed during the course of this research conformed to a stereotype that previously had been practised by the researcher and taught to students, and then evaluated positively when they perpetuated the model. The opportunity for further study and reflection enabled this author to examine the previously unchallenged method of taking a booking history.

The following recommendations are made on the basis of the findings:

Format of the booking interview

The format of the booking interview should be redesigned to enable the midwife to obtain accurately the pertinent, factual detail relevant to the woman's midwifery and obstetric care. This research showed that in the course of the nursing process interview, much relevant information was obtained that had not been gathered in the course of the traditional interview. The nursing process format also demonstrated that its use would enable a midwife to explore the woman's feelings and expectations which, as shown in this study, are relevant to the planning of her subsequent care.

Conduct of the interview

Consideration should be given to ensuring that booking interviews are undertaken by experienced midwives who work permanently in the antenatal clinic, unless a senior student midwife is gaining experience under supervision.

Midwives should introduce themselves by name and grade to women at the commencement of the interview and state that they are midwives. The purpose of the interview should be explained and questions invited at the outset.

Midwives should enquire from the woman how she wishes to be addressed. Her answer should be recorded in a prominent place on the notes for future reference.

Learning interviewing skills

Other methods of teaching booking interview skills should be explored in addition to the role-model method. Suggestions include recording and listening to play-back of the interview, listening to specimen recorded interviews, both good and bad, analysis of transcribed interviews for communication breakdown, role-play and peer-group observation and critique. When the role-model method is employed it should be ensured that the role model is an experienced midwife with a good interview technique, so that clichés and faulty styles of questioning are not perpetuated.

Interactive skills and interview technique should be included in the curriculum for student midwife training and incorporated into further education and in-service education programmes for qualified midwives and other personnel.

There is a need to improve the way in which midwives obtain information from childbearing women. Use of a nursing process assessment
and education in interview techniques would go some way to achieving
this and thereby raising the standard of midwifery care provided for
women.

APPENDIX A: SCHEDULE FOR SEMI-STRUCTURED INTERVIEW WITH INTERVIEWING MIDWIFE

Thank you for agreeing to talk to me and for allowing me to record your conversation with the mothers.

1. How long have you been working as a midwife? (What stage of training have
   you reached?)
2. How long have you been working in the antenatal clinic?
3. Is this a permanent position or do you move around the hospital?
4. What other nursing qualifications do you hold?
5. What were you taught about taking a mother's booking history while you
   were training?
6. What preparation or further teaching have you had for recording a mother's
   booking history since you have been working in clinic as a qualified midwife?
7. Do you think that further preparation or teaching is necessary for qualified
   midwives when they come to work in the antenatal clinic?
8. What teaching have you had in midwifery about interviewing skills?
9. What have you been taught in midwifery about counselling mothers?
10. What have you been taught as a midwife about giving health education and
    teaching mothers on a person-to-person basis?
11. Would you say that you had had most teaching about taking a mother's
    booking history from tutors in the school or from midwives working in the
    antenatal clinic?
12. How adequately prepared did you feel when you came to record your first
    booking history?
13. Did you record your first unsupervised booking history as a student or as a
    qualified midwife?
14. Now that you have had some experience recording mothers' booking
    histories, do you feel: very confident, confident, fairly confident, unsure, very
    unsure?
15. How do you feel about the interviews I recorded on cassette? Are there any
    comments you would like to make about your performance or the way the
    mother responded?
16. What further midwifery education or in-service training have you had to help
    you keep up to date with current developments in midwifery and obstetric
    care since you have been working in clinics?
17. To what extent has this met your needs?
18. How do/would you teach a student midwife to record a mother's booking
    history?
19. How are mothers allocated to midwives to have their booking histories
    taken?
20. Could it sometimes happen that a mother with a complicated history or
    language problem is interviewed by someone relatively inexperienced in
    recording a history?

21. Do you think a midwife is the best person to record a mother's booking history?
22. What are your reasons for thinking this?
23. What part, if any, do you think doctors should have in recording a mother's history?
24. Do doctors in this hospital duplicate any part of the booking history already recorded from the mother by a midwife?
25. To what extent do you think the booking interview enables a midwife to establish a relationship with the mother whose history she has recorded?
26. If it were possible for the mother to be cared for at every subsequent antenatal visit by the midwife who recorded her booking history, what would you consider the advantages and/or disadvantages to be?
27. What do you think about keeping a separate record of care given by a midwife to a mother during pregnancy, in addition to the Co-operation card?
28. To what extent do you think midwives are making the best possible use of the information that is currently obtained from the mother at booking clinic?
29. Is there any additional information you would like midwives to obtain from mothers at booking clinic that might enable them to give improved care to mothers in pregnancy, labour and the puerperium?
30. In your opinion, to what extent do the obstetricians in this hospital allow midwives to fulfil their role in giving antenatal care to mothers?
31. In a sentence or two, will you tell me what you know about nursing process?
32. To what extent to you think nursing process has a place in midwifery care?
33. How could you see nursing process operating in this clinic?
34. Are there any further comments you would like to make or questions you wish to ask?

Thank you for talking with me.

APPENDIX B: POST-HISTORY QUESTIONNAIRE FOR MOTHERS

1. Do you think that the person who took your history was:
   a) a doctor _____ b) a nurse _____ c) a midwife _____
   d) other (please state) _____
2. Can you identify the grade of the person who talked to you?
   a) Registrar _____ b) Sister _____ c) Staff Nurse/Midwife _____
   d) Student Nurse/Midwife _____ e) other (please state) _____
3. Do you feel the person put you at ease before they started to take your history?
   a) Yes _____ b) No _____ c) Don't know _____
4. Were any words used that were unfamiliar to you, and which you did not understand?
   a) Yes _____ b) No _____ c) Don't know _____
   If 'yes' please state what they were: _____
   _____
5. Did you feel the interviewer listened to all you had to say?
   a) Yes _____ b) No _____ c) Don't know _____
   If 'no' please state: _____
   _____
6. Did you feel that everything you said was understood by the person taking your history?

a) Yes _____ b) No _____ c) Don't know _____
7. Do you know why each question was asked?
   a) Yes _____ b) No _____ c) Don't know _____
   Please state which questions you don't know the reason for:
   _____
   _____

8. Did you feel free to ask all the questions you wanted to?
   a) Yes _____ b) No _____ c) Don't know _____
   If 'no' please state: _____
   _____

9. Is there any information you expected to receive but were not given?
   a) Yes _____ b) No _____ c) Don't know _____
   If 'yes' please state what it was: _____
   _____

10. Do you think there is anything relevant to your care in pregnancy or labour which you were not asked about?
    a) Yes _____ b) No _____ c) Don't know _____
    If 'yes' please state: _____
    _____

11. Would you describe the speed of the interview as:
    a) rushed _____ b) unhurried _____ c) long drawn-out _____
    d) other, (please state) _____

12. Is there any way in which you would have liked the booking interview to be different?
    a) Yes _____ b) No _____ c) Don't know _____
    If 'yes' please state how: _____
    _____

13. Would you say that you had formed a relationship with the person who took your history?
    a) Yes _____ b) No _____ c) Don't know _____

14. Would you like the person who took your history to care for you every time you came to antenatal clinic?
    a) Yes _____ b) No _____ c) Don't know _____

15. Are you satisfied about the way the interview ended?
    a) Yes _____ b) No _____ c) Don't know _____
    If 'no' please state why: _____
    _____

16. Please state what you understand is to happen for the rest of today's visit
    _____
    _____

17. How often should you come to antenatal clinic for the rest of your pregnancy?
    _____

18. Are there any other comments you wish to make about the history-taking interview?
    _____
    _____

Thank you very much for your help.

_____

Interviewer's code   Grade

APPENDIX C: SCHEDULE FOR STRUCTURED INTERVIEW WITH MOTHERS FOLLOWING A TRADITIONAL BOOKING INTERVIEW BASED ON OREM'S MODEL

Hospital   **Date**   **Interview Code**

I would like to ask you some further questions on topics that are not usually asked when your history is taken. Because I am not working for the hospital, I am not able to give you information, which you may not already know, about the topics we talk about. You should ask the hospital midwives to give you this. I would also like to write down all that you say, so I hope you will not find this disturbing. The more you can tell me, the more helpful it will be. Thank you.

Please would you describe your usual diet in any normal day before you became pregnant.

1a. What would you have for breakfast?
1b. What would you eat at lunchtime?
1c. What would a normal evening meal consist of?
1d. What other snacks might be taken during the day?
1e. Has there been any alteration in your usual eating pattern since you became pregnant?
1f. Do you know what food requirements are recommended during pregnancy?
2a. How much fluid would you usually drink in a 24-hour period before you became pregnant (in cups)?
2b. How much milk did you usually have each day (including that in custard or as yoghurt)?
2c. How much of your total fluid consumption in any day is alcohol?
2d. Has there been any alteration in your fluid intake or drinking pattern since the start of pregnancy?
2e. Do you know what fluid requirements are recommended when you are pregnant?
3a. Will you describe your usual pattern of daily activity (how you spend a normal day)?
3b. Do you pursue any sports or undertake any vigorous exercise?
3c. Does your job require you to stand for long periods or to be on your feet for any length of time?
3d. Have you made any changes in your activities since pregnancy began?
4a. Do you usually have any difficulty with breathing or experience any periods of breathlessness?
4b. Do you know how breathing may be affected during pregnancy?
5a. Do you usually have your bowels opened every day?
5b. Are you aware of any tendency to constipation or diarrhoea when you are not pregnant?
5c. How do you usually cope with this?
5d. Did you have any trouble with haemorrhoids before you became pregnant?
5e. Have you noticed any change with your bowels or haemorrhoids since pregnancy began?
5f. Do you usually pass urine without difficulty?
5g. Did you usually have to get up at night to go to the toilet before you became pregnant?
5h. Has there been any alteration in this pattern since you have been pregnant?

5i. Are you aware of any changes that may occur with your bladder or bowel function now that you are pregnant?

6a. How did you feel when you first realized that you were pregnant?

6b. How do you feel about being pregnant now?

6c. What have you read or what do you know about having a baby and becoming a mother?

6d. What do you think about labour and actually giving birth to the baby?

6e. How well do you think you (and your husband) will manage a new baby?

6f. What are your views about feeding the baby?

6g. Do you know how to care for your breasts during pregnancy?

6h. Do you know about the Parentcraft Classes that are provided in this hospital?

6i. Do you plan to attend these?

7a. What changes to your present lifestyle do you think pregnancy and having a baby will make for you (and your husband)?

7b. How do you feel about this?

7c. What family or other support do you have?

7d. Are there any aspects of your religious practice that might be affected when you are in hospital?

8a. Do you know what footwear and clothing are recommended while you are pregnant?

8b. Do you know how to care for your teeth and gums during pregnancy?

8c. When did you last attend a dentist, or when is your next dental appointment?

8d. Do you know things or situations you should avoid in pregnancy because they might be a hazard or a threat to you and/or your baby?

8e. Have you taken any steps to avoid such risks since pregnancy began?

8f. What things would make you contact your doctor or the hospital while you are pregnant?

8g. Is there anything that usually makes you feel stressed or anxious?

8h. Is there anything about having a baby or being a parent might do to cause you to feel stressed, anxious or embarrassed, for example?

9a. Would you say that you are the sort of person who likes a lot of people around you or do you prefer your own company?

9b. Have you ever been in hospital before as a patient?

9c. Have you ever been apart from your husband/children/family before?

9d. How do you usually react to being apart from your husband/children/family?

9e. How do they usually react to being apart from you?

9f. How do you think you will cope with being in hospital to have the baby, especially during labour?

9g. How do you think your husband will cope while you are in hospital?

9h. What is your reaction to being cared for by hospital staff and midwives whom you may not have met before?

9i. Do you have any views about student doctors or midwives looking after you while you are at the clinic or in hospital?

10a. How many hours sleep do you usually have each night?

10b. Has your sleep pattern changed at all since you have been pregnant?

10c. Do you know what rest and exercise are recommended during pregnancy?

11. Is there anything you would like to ask me?

12a. General appearance

12b. Estimate of apparent intelligence

12c. Personality

12d. Social or cultural background
12e. Language or difficulty with speech
12f. Any hearing loss, or physical feature of note

Thank you very much for your help and for letting me talk to you.

REFERENCES

Adams, M., Armstrong-Esther, C., Bryar, R., Doberley, J., Strong, G. and Ward, E. (1981) Trial run. *Nursing Mirror, 153* (15), 32–35.
Bailey, R.E. (1972) *Mayes Midwifery*, 8th edn. Bailliere Tindall, London.
Ball, J.A. (1981) The effect of present patterns of maternity care on the emotional needs of mothers, Part 3. *Midwives Chronicle, 94* (1122), 231–7.
Ball, J.A. and Stanley, J. (1984) A joint presentation – stress and the mother. *Midwives Chronicle, 79* (1162), xviii–xxii.
Birdwhistell, R.L. (1968) Kinesics. In M. Argyle (ed.) *Social encounters: Readings in social interaction*, Penguin, London.
Bowers, J., Charles, J. and Wood, R. (1987) *Nursing process in midwifery – Has it a place?* Middle management course no. 44 project, Oldham A.H.A.
Browne, J. and Dixon, G. (1978) *Browne's antenatal care*, 11th edn. English Language Book Society and Churchill Livingstone, London.
Bryans, B.A.C. (1985) The midwifery process: Does it work? *Midwives Chronicle, 98* (1173), 280.
Bryar, R. (1986) Introducing change in *Research and the Midwife Conference Proceedings, 1986.* Nursing Research Unit, King's College, University of London, London.
Bryar, R. (1987) A study of the introduction of the nursing process in a maternity unit. Unpublished M. Phil thesis, Polytechnic of the South Bank, London.
Bryar, R. and Strong, G. (1983) Trial run continued. *Nursing Mirror, 79* (41), 45–48.
Central Midwives Board (1978) *Notices concerning a midwife's Code of Practice.* C.M.B., London
Clarke, M. (1978) Getting through the work. In R. Dingwall and J. McIntosh (eds), *Readings in the sociology of nursing*, Churchill Livingstone, Edinburgh.
Dewey, J. (1910) *How we think.* Heath, Boston.
Fender, H. (1981) Midwifery care plans, *Association of Radical Midwives Newsletter, 11*, 10–12.
Flint, (1983) Antenatal clinics 6 – Using the midwifery process. *Nursing Mirror, 156* (1) 16–17.
Gibbs, J. (1983) Matter of convenience. *Nursing Mirror, 156* (2), 61–63.
Heath, J., Bradshaw, J., Law, G.M. and Whitfield, S. (1986) *Planned individualised care of mother, baby and the family unit.* English National Board. Learning Resources Unit, Sheffield.
de Julia, N. (1980) The nursing interview. *Australian Nursing Journal, 10* (5), 38–39.
Keane, J. (1982) *The nursing process applied to midwifery vols 1 and 2.* Unpublished DANS dissertation, University of Manchester.
Kitzinger, S. (1983) *New good birth guide.* Penguin, Harmondsworth.
MacLeod Clark, J. (1981) Communication in nursing. *Nursing Times, 77* (1), 12–18.

Marriner, A. (1969) *The nursing process: A scientific approach to nursing care*, 2nd edn. C.V. Mosby, St. Louis.

McGuire, P. and Rutter, D. (1976) Training medical students to communicate. In A.C. Bennett (ed.), *Communication between doctors and patients*, Nuffield Provincial Hospital Trust, Oxford University Press, Oxford.

McCain, R.F. (1965) Nursing by assessment, not intuition. *American Journal of Nursing*, *64* (4), 82–83.

Methven, R. (1986a) Care plan for a woman having antenatal care, based on Orem's self-care model. In C. Webb (ed.), *Women's health: Midwifery and gynaecological nursing*, Hodder and Stoughton, London.

Methven, R. (1986b) Care plan for a woman during pregnancy, labour and the puerperium, based on Henderson's activities-of-daily-living model. In C. Webb (ed.), *Women's health: Midwifery and gynaecological nursing*, Hodder and Stoughton, London.

Myles, M. (1981) *Textbook for midwives*, 9th edn. Churchill Livingstone, Edinburgh.

Open University (1979) Data collection procedures in research methods. In *Education and the social sciences*, Block 4, DE 304 Open University Press, Milton Keynes.

Orem, D.C. (1980) *Nursing concepts of practice*, 2nd edn. McGraw Hill, New York.

Pearson, A. and Vaughan, B. (1986) *Nursing models for practice.* Heineman, London.

Plant, M. (1986) Drinking in pregnancy and fetal harm: Results from a Scottish prospective study. *Midwifery*, *2* (2), 81–85.

Roesthilsberger, F.J. and Dickson, W.J. (1939) *Management and the worker.* Harvard University Press, Cambridge, Mass.

Robinson, J. (1978) *Documenting patient care responsibility.* Ravenswood Publications, Beckenham.

Smutts, J.C. (1926) *Key concepts for the study and practice of nursing*, 2nd edn. C.V. Mosby, St. Louis.

Thomson, A.M. (1980) Planned or unplanned – Are midwives ready for the 1980s? *Midwives Chronicle*, *93* (1106), 68–72.

Towler, J. and Butler-Manuel, R.B. (1980) *Modern obstetrics for student midwives*, 2nd edn. Lloyd-Luke, London.

Whitfield, S. (1983) 1982 Sir William Power Memorial Lecture: The midwifery process in practice. *Midwives Chronicle*, *96* (1145), 186–9.

CHAPTER FOUR

Psychosocial effectiveness of antenatal and postnatal care

Maureen Porter and Sally Macintyre

INTRODUCTION

In advice literature for expectant women there is much stress on the benefits of antenatal and postnatal care, and on the importance of attending for all scheduled check-ups. This advice literature (British Medical Association, 1975; Scottish Health Education Group, 1980; Health Education Council, 1984), and the policy literature on which it is based (e.g. British Paediatric Association/Royal College of Obstetricians and Gynaecologists, 1978; Social Services Committee, 1980) emphasizes the importance of these check-ups not only for clinical purposes, but also for providing women with advice, information and reassurance. While it has been recognized for some time (Garcia, 1982) that women may be put off by the manner in which maternity care is provided (e.g., by long waiting times, inconvenient appointment times, lack of continuity of care), the assumption that the care offered is actually beneficial, both clinically and psychosocially, is rarely questioned.

Elsewhere we have argued that this assumption should be questioned, and that there is a need to examine the effectiveness of antenatal care in relation to its various objectives (Hall, Macintyre and Porter, 1985). In this chapter we want to focus not on the clinical efficacy of antenatal and postnatal maternity care (whether it can successfully detect and treat or prevent clinical problems), but rather on its psychosocial effectiveness – whether it meets the needs of women for support, explanation, information and encouragement, during pregnancy and the puerperium. We suggest that women's experiences in antenatal and postnatal clinics often fall short of the expectations raised by the maternity advice literature. Our observations of consultations in antenatal and postnatal clinics and wards not only confirm most of the dissatisfactions with the quality of care reported by women in interview (or reported to pressure groups), but also indicate that those 'complaints' may understate rather than overstate the case.

MATERIALS AND METHODS

We base our argument on a number of studies conducted by the authors and others in Aberdeen over the past ten years. These studies have been concerned with married women's experience of first pregnancy (Macintyre, 1981), an evaluation of a new system of antenatal care introduced in Aberdeen in 1980 (Hall, Macintyre and Porter, 1985), and a study of contraceptive decision-making following obstetric events such as births, induced and spontaneous abortions (Porter, 1986). Together, these studies have involved extended periods of observation in gynaecology, antenatal and postnatal clinics; in gynaecology, labour and postnatal wards; and to a lesser extent in general practitioners' surgeries. They have also involved interviews with women at varying points in pregnancy and early motherhood. The main providers of antenatal care – obstetricians, general practitioners, midwives and health visitors – have also been interviewed at various points in time. Although some midwives' clinics were observed, there were too few to include in the analysis. Table 4.1 shows the main sources of data.

Each of these studies was concerned with women's experiences of some aspect of maternity care and was designed to examine that experience in as reliable a manner as possible. Wherever possible, we tried to triangulate our data (Denzin, 1970), for example by observing interactions in the various settings as well as interviewing women and doctors about the consultations observed. In this way we were able to obtain a number of different measures of the same phenomena, aiming thereby to increase the reliability and validity of our data. Our findings confirm and also extend those of many other researchers who have relied solely upon interview and/or questionnaire methods to obtain women's opinions of the maternity care they have received.

Gaining access to most of the settings studied was a lengthy and difficult process involving negotiation with local ethical and professional committees and individual staff. In some cases, official bodies refused to countenance a study; in others, individual staff or clinics refused to participate. In still others, junior staff were required to participate, possibly unwillingly, by their superiors. Most medical, midwifery and nursing staff said that they found our presence threatening initially but they soon adjusted and accepted it, treating us as colleagues and confidants. Women 'patients' rarely objected to our presence and in some circumstances seemed grateful for it, even addressing questions and comments to us. A few staff, however, continued to mind our presence and succeeded in making us and sometimes the women feel very uncomfortable. If, as we suspected and were often told, staff were 'on their best behaviour' because of our presence, it is worrying to consider how poor might be the interaction in consultations not observed.

Table 4.1 Sources of data on interaction in antenatal clinics

Year	Author	Description of study	Main methods	Sample
1976–80	S. Macintyre	prospective interview study of married women's expectations and experiences of first pregnancy	serial interviews at booking, 24 wks, 34 wks and postpartum	50 women
			observation of labour and delivery	17 women
1980–85	S. Macintyre et al.	before and after evaluation of new system of antenatal care introduced in Aberdeen in 1980	observation of consultant/SR antenatal clinics before, during and after the change	755 consultations
			questionnaire to clinic attenders before, during and after the change	1253 questionnaires
			interviews with expectant women after the change	232 women
			interviews with care providers – obstetricians, GPs, midwives and HVs – during and after the change	233 providers

1985–86	M. Porter	prospective study of women's contraceptive decision-making	observation of hospital wards and clinics – postnatal, antenatal and gynaecological	530 consultations
			observations of general practitioners' surgeries	282 consultations
			observation of family planning clinic sessions	132 consultations
			interviews with observed women	175 women
			interviews with observed doctors	20 doctors

Source: Compiled by the authors.

ANTENATAL CARE

Women's views on the benefits and experience of antenatal care have been elicited in a large number of recent studies (Reid and McIlwaine, 1980; O'Brien and Smith, 1981; Hall *et al.*, 1985). It has been consistently reported that they object to long waiting times; the impersonal, production-line atmosphere of most clinics; the lack of consistent information, advice and support; and the discontinuity of care providers (Garcia, 1982). It has been shown that in this they are not so different from patients attending many other sorts of medical clinics (Macintyre, 1982), communication failure being the aspect most complained of in all health care (Cartwright, 1964; Reynolds, 1978; Fitton and Acheson, 1979). These complaints are thus not peculiar to pregnant women or antenatal care.

It is because of findings such as these that improvements in the manner in which care is delivered have been suggested (and indeed implemented). Throughout Britain, attempts have been made to improve communications between pregnant and labouring women and their attendants, to reduce waiting times, to introduce more continuity of care and greater personalization, and so on (Macintyre and Porter, in press). Many of these innovations have involved changes such as wallpapering rooms, redesigning gowns, or enlarging cubicles; alternatively they have attempted to increase the quantity of care, or the status of care-providers, on the assumption that more care must be better care. In making these changes, few have questioned the actual content or benefits of care rather than the manner in which it is delivered.

An exception was the innovation introduced by the consultant obstetrician Marion Hall and her colleagues in Aberdeen. These care-providers questioned whether antenatal care really could do as much good as was supposed. They examined the case records of all women living in Aberdeen city and suburbs who delivered in Aberdeen in a one-year period (1975) in order to assess the productivity of routine antenatal visits; the problems that arise in spite of regular monitoring; and the efficiency of the present system in identifying high-risk women, detecting problems in mother and baby, and in using available resources including specialized investigations and the time of staff and of expectant women. They concluded that the benefits it is possible to achieve from routine antenatal visits had hitherto been overestimated. Many problems arose despite routine care (or could not have been predicted by routine care); others were missed or misdiagnosed (Chng *et al.*, 1980; Hall *et al.*, 1980; Hall, 1981). The researchers also learned from work undertaken locally and simultaneously that women often got little out of these visits and experienced them as unpleasant and alienating (Macintyre, 1981). As a result they designed and implemented a new system of antenatal care in which the purpose of each visit was clearly specified, the number of routine visits was reduced, and care was concentrated less than previously in the hands of specialists. It was expected that these changes would bring about a reduction in the number of women attending specialist hospital clinics, increase the time available for each woman's specialist consultation, reduce waiting times, and improve continuity of care (Hall *et al.*, 1985).

FINDINGS

The Aberdeen-based study of 50 married primigravidae, on which the Aberdeen innovators had drawn, used a series of interviews, at the time of booking, 24 and 36 weeks gestation, and postpartum, to chart the development of women's ideas and experiences of first pregnancy (Macintyre, 1981). Macintyre asked what women thought was the purpose of routine antenatal care and what benefit the women themselves got out of their antenatal visits. At this time it was the policy for all primigravidae to attend specialist hospital clinics for all their antenatal care, partly because they were seen as being at greater risk of complications and partly because a pool of primigravidae was needed for research purposes. Regardless of education, social class, reading or prior contact with the health services, the majority of Macintyre's respondents could not identify specific benefits of attending at the time of the first interview. It was something they had not really thought about or been given any information about. They went because they thought they ought to or because they believed that there must be some point, otherwise antenatal care would not exist. Their comments included the following:

> I've never thought about it, never thought about it. I just know that you have to go and that's it.

> Well, I mean they are obviously trained specially for it, there must be some point.

> I don't think we would suffer [with no antenatal care]. As I say, before you didn't have it and there was plenty of healthy babies born.... There must be a purpose, otherwise it wouldn't be there.

At later interviews women were still unable to identify specific benefits stemming from their visits, though some derived reassurance from them. At 34 weeks only 5% said their visits were useful, 82% said they were neutral or reassuring, and 13% said that they were useless:

> They haven't been much use really. It's just always better getting a check.

> The doctor comes in and he puts one hand on my belly and he goes away out again! He says, 'That's fine', and I says, 'Is that all?'

> I wouldn't like not to go, put it that way.

After the birth women were even more negative. Less than half said then that it would not have made any difference if they had been to the doctor or clinic only twice in the whole pregnancy, and a small minority said they would have been better off with less care. Those who had had a straightforward pregnancy could not see how it had helped them, while those who had had complications pointed out that it had not prevented them.

Thus, despite the emphasis on encouraging women to attend for care in order to help their baby, the majority of women studied did not believe that antenatal care would greatly benefit them or their baby, and attended because they felt it might benefit them in some unspecified way – and because they would feel guilty if it turned out that such visits might indeed be beneficial. In the later assessment of antenatal care in Aberdeen, these questions were repeated, with very similar results, with pregnant women who had experienced the new system of antenatal care. Two hundred and thirty-two women were interviewed at 36 weeks gestation. Nearly half of them (46%) said they got nothing at all out of their hospital booking visit, and a similar proportion experienced their 30-week routine hospital check-up as unpleasant, upsetting or mixed. As a result of the new system, the majority of women were attending their GPs for antenatal care and only those with special problems or unusual circumstances routinely attended the specialist clinic. The results of satisfaction scales administered to the women reflected these differences. Tables 4.2–4.6 show that women derived considerably less satisfaction from their hospital visits than from those to their GPs, whether the criterion be overall satisfaction, reassurance, benefit, enjoyment or atmosphere.

Table 4.7 shows their responses to the manner of the staff with whom they routinely came into contact. GPs and midwives were rated similarly as fairly sympathetic, while obstetricians were likely to be seen as much less sympathetic.

The health education literature exhorting women to attend for care had been successful, and despite having doubts about whether their hospital visits were doing them any good, women continued to attend.

Table 4.2 Overall satisfaction by usual place of care

Overall satisfaction	Usual place of care		
	General practitioner (n = 164) %	Hospital (n = 42) %	All (n = 206) %
dissatisfied/fairly dissatisfied	1	5	1
mixed feelings	15	12	14
satisfied/fairly satisfied	84	83	84

Source: Antenatal care study

Table 4.3 Reassurance perceived by place visited

Reassurance	Place of visit			
	General practitioner (n = 161) %	Peripheral clinic (n = 27) %	Hospital (n = 117) %	All (n = 305)* %
fairly/very anxiety-provoking	2	18	22	11
neutral/OK	9	30	30	19
fairly/very reassuring	89	52	49	70

Source: Antenatal care study
*Women who had regularly visited more than one clinic were asked about each.

Table 4.4 Perceived benefit by place visited

Benefit	Place of visit			
	General practitioner (n = 161) %	Peripheral clinic (n = 27) %	Hospital (n = 117) %	All (n = 305)* %
harmful/fairly harmful	—	11	2	2
neutral	10	26	20	15
beneficial/fairly beneficial	90	63	79	83

Source: Antenatal care study
*Women who had regularly visited more than one clinic were asked about each.

We found that very few reported missing visits, and those that did generally had very good reasons for not going (for example, illness, a sick child or lack of transportation to hospital). A clinic record of non-attenders during this period suggests that women's own reports were accurate, that is, that there were vanishingly small numbers of appointments not kept without good reason. It is simply not true, as has often been suggested, that women in Aberdeen or elsewhere are defaulting

Table 4.5 Enjoyment by place visited

Enjoyment	Place of visit			
	General practitioner (n = 161) %	Peripheral clinic (n = 27) %	Hospital (n = 117) %	All (n = 305)* %
unpleasant/fairly unpleasant	—	15	14	7
OK	47	48	66	54
enjoyable/fairly enjoyable	54	38	21	39

Source: Antenatal care study
*Women who had regularly visited more than one clinic were asked about each.

Table 4.6 Perceived atmosphere by place visited

Atmosphere	Place of visit			
	General practitioner (n = 161) %	Peripheral clinic (n = 34) %	Hospital (n = 118) %	All (n = 313)* %
cold and hostile or fairly so	3	15	10	7
OK	10	32	40	24
warm and welcoming or fairly so	87	52	50	69

Source: Antenatal care study
*Women who had regularly visited more than one clinic were asked about each.

from antenatal visits in large numbers (Social Services Committee, 1980). It might be reasonable to assume, therefore, that they continued to attend because they were obtaining some other benefit from their visits. Among those suggested by the advice literature as resulting from regular attendance are the opportunity to ask questions, raise doubts and worries, and/or discuss the progress of the pregnancy and the meaning of tests and procedures:

Table 4.7 Perceived manner of types of staff

Manner	General practitioner (n = 159) %	Obstetrician (n = 154) %	Midwife (n = 149) %
unsympathetic or fairly so	1	17	6
average	17	47	28
sympathetic or fairly so	82	35	67

Source: Antenatal care study

> Throughout your pregnancy you will have regular check-ups either at an antenatal clinic or with your own doctor. This is to make sure that you and the baby are fit and well, to check the baby is developing properly, and as far as possible to prevent anything going wrong ... These check-ups also give you a chance to get answers to the questions and worries that are bound to crop up at different stages of your pregnancy (Health Education Council, 1984).

Other literature invites women not only to mention worries but even to make a list of questions to ask at their visits:

> There may be several questions you want to ask the staff of the clinic. It's a good idea to write down any questions that occur to you before your visit so that you won't forget them when you get there. Never be afraid to ask the doctor or nurses if you don't understand something or if you have a problem that is worrying you (Scottish Health Education Group, 1980).

Our observations suggest that these incentives are not met in the context of specialist antenatal clinics (although they may be in midwives' clinics or those run by GPs). Of the women whose consultations were observed at the specialist antenatal clinic, 60% asked no questions at all, 20% asked one question, and 20% asked more than one question. Often these questions concerned routine administrative matters such as maternity benefits or where to book a bed, but they also included the progress of the pregnancy, size or lie of the baby, and other topics that one would have expected to be covered routinely in the consultation. In 60% of hospital consultations observed, there was no discussion at all of topics other than those basic subjects of question-and-answer format that are essential for the main clinical purpose of the consultation, for example, date of last period, first experience of movements, symptoms and so on. Additional topics and some of the conventions for coding them are shown in Figure 4.1. These topics included subjects of antenatal advice or education, information or advice about minor or major morbidity, and explanations of conditions or procedures. As we adopted a very liberal definition of topics (for example, 'Do you smoke? No', was counted as discussion of smoking), it was disquieting to find that in only 40% of the consultations were any topics discussed at all and that in half

Figure 4.1 Topics discussed in antenatal consultations: list of those to be included, and conventions for including them.

1. Breast feeding (even if only just asks re intentions)
2. Smoking (even if just comments)
   Rest at home/stopping work (asks if getting enough rest or advises her to rest)
4. Diet/weight control (advice about taking off or putting on weight or whether weight gain is OK. *Not* sufficient if Dr just says 'weight OK' or 'have you put on more than last time' etc. (i.e. *not* in ref. to intra uterine growth retardation)
5. Future contraceptive plans (including female or male sterilization. *Not* including past contraception where this appears only to establish her dates during this pregnancy)
6. Dental health
7. Social (adoption, marriage, marriage breakdown, etc.)
8. PP depression/depression/mood changes
9. Sexual behaviour (whether OK to have sex, to abstain from it, when to resume it)

Pregnancy related morbidity

10. Varicose veins	*not* to be included if patient mentions them but nothing said/done in response.
11. Nausea/vomiting	
12. Heartburn/indigestion	to *be* included if doctor asks about them.
13. Faintness/dizziness	*not* to be included if doctor's questions relate
14. Cramp	only to establishing gestation and not to
15. Backache	helping/advising women.
16. Pain	cramp/backache/pain *not* to be included
17. Constipation	if questions relate to whether any signs of labour.

(i.e. excluding vaginal discharge, anaemia if just iron, fetal movements, BP, contractions, proteinuria, urinary tract infection)
18. Other concurrent morbidity, e.g. sore throat, rash, breathlessness, etc. (with some exclusions as above, e.g. vaginal discharge)
19. Other advice about do's, don'ts – sports, travelling, relaxation classes, alcohol, drug ingestion, housework, etc.
20. Discussion about procedures and what they entail (e.g. amniocentesis, episiotomy, induction)
21. Discussion about conditions and their implications (e.g. breech, PET, placenta praevia, etc.)

of these only one topic featured. The topics that were discussed are shown in Table 4.8, which reveals that infant feeding, smoking and rest were the most common topics raised.

It might be argued that women asked so few questions because topics of interest or importance to them were already being covered in the discussion anyway. But this seemed not to be the case. Of the women seeing obstetricians, 45% neither asked any questions nor had any topics discussed with them. Even when invited by the doctor to ask any questions they wished, relatively few women did so. Yet when they were interviewed later about the hospital consultation, an alarming 50% said that they had had questions they wished to ask but were too inhibited to do so, were put off by the doctor's attitude or behaviour, lacked the opportunity, or forgot in the excitement of the event.

Consultant clinics seem to be structured in such a way that women rarely have an opportunity to ask questions or raise any doubts they may have. The following examples are typical of routine 34- and 40-week check-ups for women having 'shared care'.

Table 4.8 Topics discussed in antenatal consultations

Topic	Number of mentions	Consultations where mentioned %
infant feeding	16	9.3
smoking	16	9.3
rest	15	8.7
diet/weight	9	5.2
social/depression/sex	8	4.7
varicose veins	8	4.7
contraception	7	4.1
backache	5	2.9
dental	3	1.8
nausea/vomiting	4	2.3
heartburn/indigestion	4	2.3
pain	3	1.8
faintness/dizziness	2	1.2
other morbidity	13	7.6
dos and don'ts	2	1.2
explanation of procedure	6	3.5
explanation of condition	4	2.3
	(125)	
all consultations included	171	100%

Source: Antenatal care study.

Doctor walks in:
Doctor (reading notes): Your first baby was 3540 (referring to weight at birth, in grams). Are you keeping OK?
Woman: Yes.
Doctor (palpating): Is the baby kicking around?
Woman: Yes, all on one side. It only seems to kick here.
Doctor: Well, the baby's well grown; all the measurements are normal and satisfactory. There don't seem to be any problems. [leaving] I'll see you in six weeks.

Doctor enters.
Doctor: How are you doing?
Woman: Fine.
Doctor (palpating): You're not having any problems and you're not going into labour yet?
Woman: No, no signs of it.
Doctor: I'll give you a date to come in, say five or six days.
Woman: Yes, I was hoping you'd take me in and start me off.
Doctor gives patient a date and leaves.

Such consultations take only a minute or two. Obviously, many consultations are more complex and take much longer. But in 1982, after the new improved antenatal care system had been in operation for 18 months, the average length of time a woman spent with a specialist was still only five minutes (although individual doctors varied between four and eight minutes per woman). During this time a large number of tasks was usually accomplished. The doctor read the notes and checked them for the results of weight and blood pressure, which had usually been measured by the midwife before his or her arrival; supervised any students and residents; palpated the woman's uterus; checked for oedema, and performed any other examinations needed such as chest or pelvic examinations, repeat blood pressure, venepuncture, swabs, samples, and so on. Often the only opportunity women had to ask questions was when the doctor was writing up notes, palpating them or leaving the room to go to the next woman. An alarming proportion of seemingly important questions (e.g. where they were booked to have their baby and whom they should attend for antenatal care) was asked as the doctor was leaving the room.

Women had to ask these questions because so little was usually said during the consultation. For every doctor who gave women a choice of place for confinement – hospital or maternity home – and antenatal care – hospital clinic or 'shared care' – there was a doctor who gave them no choice or told them nothing. Surprisingly, the following examples are both of hospital booking visits:

Doctor (entering): How are you?
Woman: Fine.
Student (taking blood pressure): 120/70.

Doctor: Seventeen weeks. Ah, I see you're in some doubt about this. You have a funny cycle. Due 16th October minus three plus something. That makes you 25th September.
Doctor (examines and takes blood): This is just for routine tests. So that's you due at the end of ...
Woman: September.
Doctor: Good, right. Go to Holburn clinic in six weeks.

Doctor (reading) comments that it is the patient's second pregnancy and asks how she has been. She replies that she has had some abdominal pain and has had it ever since she had to rest at nine weeks with a threatened miscarriage. Patient says pains are especially severe at night. Doctor asks about last menstrual period (LMP) and whether patient has had any bleeding since. Doctor palpates, checks ankles and listens to chest. Doctor tells patient that she is not far enough on for alpha-feto-protein (AFP). Doctor tells her the pregnancy is going nicely and asks her to point to the site of the pain. Doctor asks if she had it during her last pregnancy. Doctor asks where she lives and writes chit (for confinement booking). Doctors tells patient to go to her GP next week for her AFP and to return to hospital clinic in 15 weeks.

Obviously, doctors are not always in a position to give women a choice of place of confinement or care but that is no justification for them not explaining the reasons for their clinical decisions.

We observed that women often mentioned things to the midwife before the doctor's arrival, and if it was appropriate, the midwife would then prompt the woman to ask the doctor, or mention it herself in some cases. It was particularly common for midwives to mention women's symptoms:

Doctor (palpating): Yes, that feels about 21 weeks.
Midwife: She had a little spotting in June.
Doctor: After intercourse?
Woman: Yes.
Midwife: She'd like a 48-hour discharge.
Doctor: Did you discuss that with your own GP?
Woman: Yes.
Midwife: Her nearest clinic is Torry.
Doctor: OK, I think that all your wishes can be granted.

Doctor says that as this is her third baby she must be well-practised at mothering, then reads aloud from notes that she has had two years of depression. Midwife interjects that she has had no treatment for it and has not even reported it to her doctor. Doctor then discusses how woman experiences it and suggests she may be the kind of person to worry about everything.

As doctor palpates, midwife says that the woman is 'terrified' because she has heard of the terrible things that doctors do at the Maternity Hospital.

(It is questionable, of course, whether the latter two women would in fact have welcomed the midwife's intervention.)

We also noticed that women who did ask questions were more likely than those who did not to be asked if they had any more questions they wished to ask:

> Woman (while doctor is writing in her notes): Is this where I get the form to apply for a maternity grant?
> Doctor answers and then says: Is there anything else you'd like to ask me?
> Woman: No, only, can my husband be there?
> Doctor: Yes, he can be there provided it's straightforward and there are no complications.

> Woman (anticipating that doctor is going to arrange next visit): Can I have my next appointment in five weeks because that's when I finish work?
> Doctor answers and then says: Any problems at all? Anything you want to ask me about?
> Woman: Oh, I do have but I forget them when I come here.
> Doctor: You should write them down, you always forget.

A few specialists invited women, particularly those who had asked no questions when invited to do so, to list them for their next visit. This is perhaps unfortunate as there was no guarantee that the woman would see the same doctor at her next visit and some hospital doctors were not so receptive to lists of questions. We observed that women who asked several questions were sometimes met with a hostile reception or patronizing tolerance and, unbeknownst to them, labelled neurotic, troublesome or insecure.

> Woman: I thought you might start me off and let me try labour?
> Doctor: No.
> Woman: And if I do start myself off will I be able to go out in 48 hours?
> Doctor: It depends on the baby's condition.
> Woman: What's the normal time people stay in for?
> Doctor: Six days.
> Woman: And what about a section?
> Doctor: That's about eight days.
> Later the woman asked: Can you have a third baby after two sections?
> Outside the consulting room the doctor commented to the researcher: Oh Lord these doctors wives!

Another described physicians' wives as 'a menace' because they fussed too much and asked too many questions.

It may be that women did not avail themselves of the opportunity to ask questions of obstetricians because they asked any questions they had of others whom they were perhaps seeing more frequently. Certainly this was what women thought, as can be seen from Table 4.9. This table is based on the responses of women interviewed for the evaluative study of antenatal care. It suggests that while women attending hospital antenatal clinics are relatively likely to ask questions of the midwife chaperoning them at the consultation, those receiving 'shared care' are more likely to save their questions for meetings with GPs. Observations of consultations in alternative settings, however, do not confirm this impression. Table 4.10 is based on the study of contraception in Scotland (Porter, 1986) and

Table 4.9 Who was asked questions by usual place of care

Who was asked	Usual place of care		
	General practitioner (n = 86) %	*Hospital (n = 63)* %	*All (n = 149)* %
GP	50	27	40
obstetrician	20	17	19
midwife/health visitor	8	19	13
more than one	20	33	26
other	2	3	3

Source: Antenatal care study.

Table 4.10 Percentage of patients who asked any questions

Patient type	*Observed (n = 392)* %	*Interviewed (n = 160)* %
hospital patients (gynae, antenatal, postnatal)	42	52
GP patients (family planning, antenatal, postnatal only)	34	45
family planning clinic patients	46	47
all patients	42	47

Source: Contraception study (Porter, 1986).

shows there to be a discrepancy between the number of women observed to ask questions and the number who recollect having asked questions when interviewed a short time later. Not only do women in fact ask their GPs fewer questions than they think they do, but they in fact ask GPs fewer questions than they ask their obstetricians.

On the other hand, women felt freer to raise topics of concern to them with GPs and family planning clinic doctors than they did with specialists, as can be seen from Table 4.11.

Conventions for coding patient-initiated topics are shown in Fig. 4.2. It was relatively easy to code these data in this manner as they had been collected with analysis of patient-initiated topics in mind. (It was not possible to recode the antenatal care study observations in this way because they had not been collected with a view to such an analysis and may even have omitted patient-initiated topics which were not relevant to antenatal care.) As GPs' antenatal consultations averaged ten minutes and the doctor usually needed only to glance at the notes in order to familiarize him or herself with the case, there seemed plenty of opportunity for women to raise any topics they wished. Many women did so, often raising topics not really relevant to the consultation, such as their job prospects or the health of relatives. As such topics also featured in family planning clinic consultations, it may be that raising a topic satisfied any need they had for information or advice and thereby appeared to the woman as a question answered. This may partly account for the discrepancy between observed and reported behaviour.

Obstetricians' responses to the questions women did ask were not always as helpful and sympathetic as might have been hoped. Although the majority of women said in interview that their questions had been answered to their satisfaction, we observed that doctors often lacked comprehension of women's difficulties and dismissed their worries, were patronizing, or apparently unable to explain the meaning of complex

Table 4.11 Patient-initiated topics by patient type

Number of topics raised	Patient type		
	Hospital	General practitioner	Family Planning clinic
	(n = 80)	(n = 83)	(n = 78)
	%	%	%
none	53	35	28
one	33	28	36
more than one	15	37	38

Source: Contraception study (Porter, 1986).

Figure 4.2 Patient-initiated additional topics.

A patient-initiated topic is one raised spontaneously by the patient which is over and above topics raised by the patient when establishing the primary purpose of the consultation. For example, in a consultation about contraception in which the patient mentions headaches, the latter will be coded but not the former (the primary purpose of the consultation having been agreed in advance of coding by discussions between the two observer/coders in which absolute accuracy is less important than consistency).

Though it should not be the main purpose of the consultation, a patient-initiated topic can be related to it; for example, symptoms mentioned by a pregnant woman attending for antenatal care. Each symptom or item should be treated as a separate topic.

A patient-initiated topic can be elicited by a question, comment or invitation from the doctor or nurse but should not be merely a factual/informative reply to the doctor or nurse. For example, the doctor asks what method of contraception postnatal patient requires. Her reply, 'The pill', is not coded but her additional statement that she is not happy because she has had problems with it in the past, is coded.

It can take the form of a question, but should not be mere clarification of something the doctor says or does. For example, the doctor says patient has a vaginal discharge; the patient asks what it is. The doctor tells woman to come back; the woman asks when or where.

If in doubt, code as a topic and discuss.

Most common topics
symptoms associated with presenting condition or other symptoms
fear/dislike of VEs, smears, venepuncture or other examinations
lifestyle, diet, weight control, smoking
own or others' mental/psychological states, e.g. depression
queries about condition, procedure, diagnosis, etc.
administrative matters, e.g. change of address, certificates

---

medical terms in simple language. The following quotations illustrate our point:

> Doctor: Go and see your doctor next week, and I'll give you a date, I think ten days over if you've not come off by then.
> Woman has not understood what giving her a date means, looks mystified and asks: When do you think the baby will come?
> Doctor: I think it might be like your previous one, which was what, term plus seven.
> He then writes in the notes.
> Woman: Will you induce the baby, or what will happen?
>
> Doctor asks if woman is due on 4th July and whether anything exciting has happened to her. Comments that her BP (blood

pressure) is up and that she has already gained as much weight as she should for the whole pregnancy. He palpates and checks ankles and tells her that she is in fact 'disgustingly normal' and quite boring and he had been hoping for a nice exciting first visit, not a boring return. Woman looks slightly offended.

Doctor (palpating): Well, I can't feel anything that shouldn't be there and the scar seems quite plastic. But I would like to get a scan done to confirm those dates. Do you know what a scan is?
Woman: Yes.
Doctor: Where do you live?
Woman tells him and says: I've had a bit of bleeding as well. Just some spots now and again. I told my own doctor about it and he said it was nothing to worry about but to tell you about it anyway.
Doctor: We'll try to get the scan done today but they're pretty busy there. Come back here at 34 weeks but go every month to your own doctor.
Doctor sent patient away without returning to the subject of her bleeding.

It was relatively common for doctors not to respond to certain topics that women raised. As in the above example, these were very often symptoms or worries that the woman was experiencing but which the doctor seemed not to deem relevant to the consultation. It was noted during observations in gynaecology clinics that the same doctors used similar strategies on patients there who raised sexual problems, infertility, or other matters not strictly relevant to the purpose of the consultation. Yet most of them felt free to raise topics that women might not define as relevant to the consultation. The following quotations come from observations in gynaecology and antenatal clinics:

> The doctor reads aloud that a patient requesting a termination of pregnancy came off the pill because she was not in a steady relationship and was not very good at remembering it. He tells her he still will not agree to sterilize her because she is too young and is separated. He asks her how she manages with four children on social security benefits. He tells her to buy children's clothes from Oxfam and not to be too proud.

> Doctor (reading): I see you're 35 now and you had your last baby in Fonthill in 1968. Why are you having another one now?
> Woman: Mind your own business.
> Doctor: Quite right.

It was very rare indeed for a woman to put a doctor in his place in this way, and rarer still for the doctor to concede the point. Later in the consultation, the doctor asked whether she and her husband were 'chuffed' with themselves and, learning that they were, satisfied his curiosity.

With such unsatisfactory interactions in antenatal clinics, it would not be surprising if women complained about them. Yet half of the 232 women interviewed about their experiences of the new system of antenatal care were satisfied with the information they had received on the progress of the pregnancy and the results of tests and examinations, and 56% were satisfied with the explanations they had been given of medical staff's activities during routine visits. Despite the paucity of health information and advice, only 26% wanted more, and such stated desires were more common among women having their first baby and those with a previous 'wasted' pregnancy. In most cases they wanted advice on what they called 'lots of little things', particularly diet, exercise and rest.

These observational data show that interaction in hospital antenatal clinics is often very poor and any criticisms of clinics and doctors that women make in interviews are not only justified but very mild. Indeed, without such observational data we might not have been aware of the gap between promise and performance and might have been misled by women's apparent satisfaction into believing that the content of care did not need changing. Most measures of satisfaction with medical care, unreliable though they may be, show patients to be fairly satisfied despite these experiences (Fitzpatrick and Hopkins, 1983; Porter and Macintyre, 1984).

POSTNATAL CARE

Unfortunately, our observations suggest that it would be appropriate to draw the same sorts of conclusions about hospital postnatal care. In hospital postnatal clinics and on postnatal wards (studied in Porter 1986), women appeared to be given contradictory information and advice, particularly about childcare and breast feeding. They seemed also to be deprived of the opportunity to ask questions or to raise any doubts or worries, and there was often little discussion of procedures or options. For example, breast feeding women were often told to use the progesterone-only pill but not why. Discussion of contraceptive choices often took place in a large, crowded ward with the doctor asking the woman from the end of her bed. The most personal matters were discussed in public as though the staff concurred in the view expressed by many women themselves that 'you leave your modesty at the door of the maternity hospital'. It is not surprising, therefore, that postnatal women were the least likely of the women observed to ask any questions. Only 28% of those observed did so, and most of these questions were asked at the 6-week postnatal check-up rather than on the ward.

At postnatal clinics, even those in general practices run by family doctors, there seemed to be a preoccupation with form-filling and physical well-being to the exclusion of the woman's feelings about her body or her baby. Several women mentioned sexual problems but these were merely noted on the form without further comment. Though the majority of those observed mentioned their excessive tiredness, doctors only took up the point if there was a posibility of anaemia. Breast feeding problems were mentioned by several women but not explored by doctors undertaking postnatal examinations. It may be that they did not feel personally qualified to assist; but they could have referred the woman to someone, perhaps a midwife or a health visitor, better able to help.

These experiences of postnatal care are not at all what women are led to expect by the advice literature on having a baby, which implies they will be treated with care and concern and will have an opportunity to raise their problems and doubts:

> Six weeks or so after the birth your doctor at the hospital should give you a complete check-up to make sure everything is back to normal. It's a good time to ask for advice on any problem you have, like tiredness or depression (Scottish Health Education Group, 1980).

> You will have a chance to talk with a doctor. Ask all the questions you want to. It is a good opportunity to sort out any problems or worries. The doctor will probably ask you whether you still have any vaginal discharge, and whether you have had a period yet. You will also be able to talk about contraception (Health Education Council, 1984).

This suggests that women are also being enticed to the postnatal clinics on false pretenses. Whether this lack of attention to women and their feelings has implications for the quality of parenthood and childcare remains to be seen. Certainly it seems likely to affect the woman's experience of parenting and possibly her ability to cope with the stresses parenthood imposes.

CONCLUSIONS

Our studies lead us to believe that campaigns aimed at enticing women to attend for antenatal and postnatal care are often misdirected. Women already do attend (often at great inconvenience) despite their occasional dissatisfaction with aspects of maternity care. The 'problem' is not high rates of defaulting, but the quality of care offered.

It is clear from our interviews as well as from the professional literature that obstetricians, GPs and midwives assent to the proposition that one function of antenatal care is to give women information, support and encouragement. In our interviews with obstetricians in Aberdeen about the new system of antenatal care, one of the reservations frequently voiced was that in reducing the number of scheduled antenatal visits, the new system was reducing opportunities for meeting these psychosocial and educational needs. Yet our observations, as well as numerous other interview-based studies (Graham and McKee, 1979; Reid and McIlwaine, 1980; O'Brien and Smith, 1981), show that consultations in antenatal and postnatal clinics often fail to provide the sort of psychosocial benefits that both professionals and clients feel should be offered.

We are therefore not suggesting that obstetricians willfully and knowingly withhold information, fail to explain tests or decisions or ignore reports of problems or requests for information. Rather, there may be features of medical training on the one hand, and of task-oriented specialist hospital clinics on the other, that render good doctor/patient communications difficult. Rather than blaming women for not attending for scheduled care, more attention should be devoted to ensuring that the care they are offered when they do attend is beneficial, both clinically and psycho-socially. Although it may be distressing to the professionals involved, one mechanism for doing this is to show from direct observations what is actually done and said in interactions with clients — which may be very different from what the professionals perceive themselves to be saying and doing.

In a book focusing primarily on the implications of research for midwifery, it is appropriate to raise the question of how far the psycho-social effectiveness of antenatal and postnatal care would be improved if midwives were to be given a greater role. Unfortunately, we have not been able to observe sufficient midwife-based care to reach any con-clusions on this. Though midwife clinics did form part of the new system of antenatal care in Aberdeen, an administrative anomaly meant that few women attended them (Hall, Macintyre and Porter, 1985). It is important not to assume that because midwives or women are providing care, it will necessarily be better than that provided by doctors or men. What is needed is a commitment to establish antenatal and postnatal clinics run by midwives and their systematic comparison with those run by doctors.

REFERENCES

British Medical Association (1975) *You and your baby Part I: Pregnancy to birth.* Family Doctor Publications, London.

British Paediatric Association/Royal College of Obstetricians and Gynaecologists (1978) Recommendations for the improvement of infant care during the perinatal period in the United Kingdom. BPA, London. Subsequently published in vol. 2 of *2nd report from the Social Services Committee Session 1979–80* (Short Report), HMSO, London, 1980.

Cartwright, A. (1964) *Human relations and hospital care.* Routledge and Kegan Paul, London.

Chng, P., Hall, M. and MacGillivray, I. (1980) An audit of antenatal care: the value of the first antenatal visit. *British Medical Journal, 281,* 1184–86.

Denzin, N. (1970) *The research act: A theoretical introduction to sociological methods.* Aldine, Chicago.

Fitton, F. and Acheson, H. (1979) *The doctor/patient relationship: A study in general practice.* HMSO, London.

Fitzpatrick, R. and Hopkins, A. (1983) Problems in the conceptual framework of patient satisfaction research: An empirical exploration. *Sociology of Health and Illness, 5* (3), 297–311.

Garcia, J. (1982) Women's views of antenatal care. In Enkin, M., and Chalmers, I. (eds), *Effectiveness and satisfaction in antenatal care,* Spastics International Medical Publications/Heinemann, London.

Graham, H. and McKee, L. (1979) *The first months of motherhood.* Report of a
    Health Education Council Project concerned with women's experiences of
    pregnancy, childbirth and the first six months. York University, mimeo.
Hall, M. (1981) Is antenatal care really necessary? *The Practitioner, 225,* 1253.
Hall, M., Chng, P. and MacGillivray, I. (1980) Is routine antenatal care worth-
    while? *Lancet, 2,* 78–80.
Hall, M., Macintyre, S. and Porter, M. (1985) *Antenatal care assessed.* Aberdeen
    University Press, Aberdeen.
Health Education Council (1984) *The pregnancy book,* HEC, London.
Macintyre, S. (1981) *Expectations and experiences of first pregnancy.* Institute of
    Medical Sociology Occasional Paper no. 5, University of Aberdeen.
Macintyre, S. (1982) Communications between pregnant women and their medi-
    cal and midwifery attendants. *Midwives Chronicle and Nursing Notes*
    (November), 387–94.
Macintyre, S. and Porter, M. (in press) Prospects and problems in promoting
    effective care at the local level. In Enkin, M., Keirse, M. and Chalmers, I.
    (eds), *Effective care in pregnancy and childbirth,* Oxford University Press,
    Oxford.
O'Brien, M. and Smith, C. (1981) Women's views and experiences of antenatal
    care. *The Practitioner, 225,* 123–25.
Porter, M. and Macintyre, S. (1984) What is, must be best: A research note on
    conservative or deferential responses to antenatal care provision. *Social
    Science and Medicine, 19* (11), 1197–1200.
Porter, M. (1986) *Free to choose? A study of contraceptive decision making.*
    Report of FPA-sponsored prospective study in Scotland. Aberdeen Uni-
    versity, mimeo.
Reid, M. and McIlwaine, G. (1980) Consumer opinion of a hospital antenatal
    clinic. *Social Science and Medicine, 14* (149), 363–68.
Reynolds, M. (1978) No news is bad news: Patients' views about communication
    in hospital. *British Medical Journal, i,* 1673–76.
Scottish Health Education Group (1980) *The book of the child,* SHEG,
    Edinburgh.
Social Services Committee (1980) Second report from the Social Services
    Committee (Chairman R. Short) session 1979–80. *Perinatal and neonatal
    mortality,* vol. 1. HMSO, London.

CHAPTER 5

Placental grading as a test of fetal well-being

Jean Proud

BACKGROUND TO THE STUDY

The appearance of the placenta on ultrasound examination changes with advancing gestational age. Four stages (grades 0–3) of placental development were first described by Grannum *et al.* (1979) in relation to fetal lung maturity. Subsequent writers have suggested that the usefulness of placental grading in this respect is limited (Quinlan *et al.*, 1982a; Hill *et al.*, 1983) whereas others have suggested an association with obstetric problems, particularly when the mature stage is reached fairly early in the pregnancy. For example, Quinlan *et al.* (1982b), Grannum and Hobbins, (1982) and Kazzi *et al.* (1983) have suggested that early maturation can be associated with maternal hypertension, intra-uterine growth retardation and fetal distress in labour.

While involved in routine ultrasound scanning at Peterborough Maternity Unit from 1979 onwards, I came to believe that early maturation of the placenta did have an association with fetal problems in labour. Early fetal maturation also seemed to have an association with women who smoke. A small retrospective study was therefore carried out in 1982 involving 277 women. They were scanned at 36 weeks gestation and the placenta was graded, using the system developed by Grannum *et al.* (1979) (see Fig. 5.1). The four grades are as follows:

Grade 0
Characteristics of this grade are: the chorionic plate is smooth, the placental substance is homogeneous, and the base layer has no echogenic areas.

Grade 1
Characteristics of this grade are: the chorionic plate becomes undulated in appearance, and the placental substance starts to contain echogenic lineai areas randomly dispersed.

Grade 2
Characteristics of this grade are: the chorionic plate becomes more indented, forming a scalloped appearance; the echogenic areas increase,

Figure 5.1 Placental grading (grade 0 to grade 3).

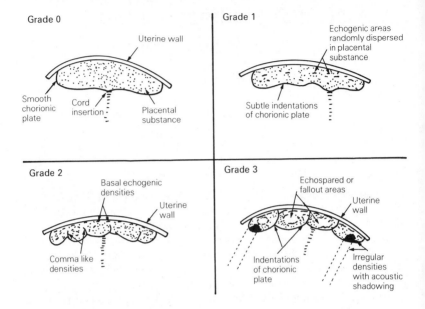

Source: Reproduced from Grannum, P.A., Berkowitz, R.L. and Hobbins, J.C. (1979) *American Journal of Obstetrics and Gynecology, 133*, 915–22.

become larger and more numerous; and the base of the placenta becomes echogenic, that is, it appears to have areas separate from the uterine wall.

Grade 3

Characteristics of this grade are: the placenta gives the appearance of being divided into the cotyledons. Within these shapes are echogenic areas varying in size and shape. The basal layer is completely echogenic, giving the appearance of 'hanging in space'.

The results of the retrospective study are shown in Table 5.1.

Two important associations were noted in this study:

1. Relatively early maturation of the placental texture, that is, to grades 2–3, appeared more frequently in women who smoked.
2. Women who showed signs of early placental maturation were much more likely to develop complications in labour.

These findings, combined with the fact that the obstetricians were beginning to use placental gradings in their clinical management, led to a decision to conduct a prospective study. This decision was taken following consultations with the staff of the National Perinatal Epidemiology

Table 5.1 Placental grading by fetal distress in labour

Placental grading	Fetal distress		
	Present	*Absent*	*Total*
Grade 3	9	2	11
Grades 0–2	5	261	266
Total	14	263	277

Sensitivity = 64%; specificity = 99%; prevalence = 5%; positive predictive value = 82%.

Note Sensitivity and specificity are measures of test accuracy. Sensitivity is the probability that a diseased patient tests positive; in this example, 9 of the 14 women with fetal distress had a grade 3 placenta, that is 64%. Specificity is the probability that a non-diseased patient tests negative; in this example, 261 of the 263 women without fetal distress did not have a grade 3 placenta, that is 99%. Prevalence refers to the percentage of patients in the study with the disease; in this example, 14 of the 277 women had fetal distress, that is 5%. Positive predictive value refers to the probability that the test predicts the presence of the disease; in this example, 9 of the 11 women with a grade 3 placenta had fetal distress, that is 82%. For further information and discussion about these measures, the reader is referred to Ingelfinger *et al.* (1987).

Unit (NPEU) in Oxford. The study had two main objectives. The first was to investigate in a randomized controlled trial whether clinical actions taken on the basis of placental grading improved perinatal outcome. A randomized controlled trial had not been undertaken before and earlier studies had been based on small populations, producing inconclusive results. The second objective, using observational data from the trial, was to test the hypothesis that early placental maturation, possibly related to maternal smoking, is a prediction of subsequent obstetric problems.

Members of the National Perinatal Epidemiology Unit supervised the project, helping with its design and with analysis of findings. Each consultant at Peterborough Maternity Unit was interviewed by myself and members of the NPEU and the nature of the trial explained to them. Their full co-operation in the conduct of the trial was assured. The Director of Nursing Services (Midwifery) was approached and permission was given that I and members of the ultrasound department and antenatal clinic could conduct the trial.

PREPARATION FOR AND DESIGN OF THE STUDY

Extensive discussion took place with NPEU regarding the design of the trial, its length and assistance needed in terms of staffing and funding.

The following issues had to be considered.

1. the amount of disruption it would cause the department
2. the increase in workload to members of staff
3. the trial design and sample size needed for it to be statistically significant.
4. the length of time the trial should take
5. the analyses to be carried out
6. ethical considerations
7. costing

Minimizing disruption to the unit

It was agreed that to cause the least inconvenience to the unit, the trial should be incorporated into the screening programme already in progress. At that time, every woman attending the consultant unit at Peterborough Maternity Unit (PMU) was scanned routinely three times during pregnancy. The first time was at the first booking visit, usually during the first trimester. This established gestational age, eliminated possibilities of multiple pregnancy or the presence of uterine and abdominal masses. The fetus was examined for abnormalities. The findings of this scan were written directly on the woman's case notes and a record card was made out for departmental use. All subsequent scans were recorded in the notes and on the card.

Two follow-up scans were performed in the last trimester, one between 30–32 weeks gestation and another at 34–36 weeks gestation, to screen for intra-uterine growth retardation. The fetal head and abdominal circumferences were measured and the ratio noted. The placenta was localized and the liquor volume assessed. The results were recorded as before. It was envisaged that placental grading would be incorporated at this stage, that is, during any scan performed in the last trimester commencing at the 30–32 weeks routine scan.

Assistance with the workload

A midwife was employed on a part-time basis as a research assistant to help with the workload and with the process of data collection. A midwife was preferred to a clerical assistant because of the need for some obstetric knowledge when collecting data.

Trial design

At the time of the 32-week scan (or the first scan thereafter), all women booked for delivery would be randomly divided into two groups. For one of these, the 'revealed group', the placental grading would be repeated for all ultrasound examinations thereafter, recorded in the notes and therefore made known to the clinician responsible for care. For the other, the 'concealed group', the placentae would be graded but the results kept in the ultrasound department and not recorded in the case notes. Subjects would retain their allocation for the remainder of their pregnancy.

Sample size

To allow for statistically significant findings, a sample size of approximately 3600, or at least 1800 women in each group of the trial (revealed and concealed), was calculated to be necessary (see Table 5.1). In 1982 there were 3328 deliveries at PMU which meant that intake to the trial would take approximately 18 months to two years.

Comparison measurements

Three groups of measurements were made to compare the two trial groups: descriptive assessments, clinical management and outcome measures.

The first were used to describe the women who were entered into the trial and assess the comparability of the randomly allocated groups in terms of:

maternal age
marital status
parity
social class
smoking habits

Aspects of clinical management assessed the impact of reporting ultrasound placental grading on subsequent clinical management including:

repeat ultrasound scan (USS) examinations
other placental function tests performed
antenatal admissions (plus length of stay)
induction of labour (plus indications)
specified abnormal fetal heart rate patterns in labour
diagnosis of fetal distress during labour
elective caesarean section (plus indications)
mode of delivery (plus indication, if operative)

Outcome measures were used to assess the relationship between placental maturation and fetal and maternal outcome, and between knowledge of ultrasound placentral grading and fetal and maternal outcome. These included:

quality of liquor during labour
Apgar score at 1 minute
Apgar score at 5 minutes
endotracheal intubation
admission (plus length of stay and indications) to special care baby unit

birthweight for gestational age
neonatal and perinatal death

Data collection

All data were collected after the woman was discharged home from hospital following delivery. Details of the scan findings would be transcribed from the departmental records, and the process and outcome data from the case notes. The data were transcribed commercially into computer-readable form and sent to NPEU staff for analysis.

Observation analyses

Two observations analyses were also performed. First, maternal smoking in pregnancy was related to the placental appearance at 32 and 36 weeks. For this analysis data from all subjects in the trial were used. Secondly, observations on women in the concealed group of the trial were used to evaluate the test 'in isolation' by relating placental appearance at 32 and 36 weeks gestation to the various measures of outcome about which information was collected for the trial. Hence the ability of placental grading to predict pregnancy outcome would be investigated further.

Randomized controlled trial

The main hypothesis to be tested in the randomized controlled trial was that knowledge of the ultrasound placental grading from 32 weeks gestation would lead to clinical action that reduced the number of babies (who were not lethally malformed) who:

1. die between the time of entry into the ultrasound examination trial and the end of the first week of life, or
2. have an Apgar score of less than 4 at 1 minute, or
3. have an Apgar score of less than 7 at 5 minutes, or
4. are admitted to the special care baby unit.

Pilot study

The first 500 intakes into the trial would be used as a pilot study.

Funding

As funding was required for a project of this size, an estimate was prepared. I had never been involved in a project such as this and I found it very difficult to make estimates. The salary for the part-time assistant was easily estimated with the help of the finance department of my own health authority. Printing costs, costs of using the computer at the National Perinatal Epidemiology Unit, Oxford, and stationery were also fairly easy to assess, but it was very difficult to know how much to budget for incidentals such as postage, telephone calls and travel.

The first source of funding explored was the Maws' Midwives Scholarship, which is awarded annually to a midwife to undertake a research project. It is awarded by Maws' in collaboration with the Royal College of Midwives and I was fortunate enough to be granted this award in 1983. The second source of funding was the Regional Health Authority. A protocol was submitted for consideration to the East Anglian Regional Health Authority together with an estimate of costs. They agreed to supply the funds needed to complete the trial.

Ethical considerations

It was hoped that in the course of this trial no woman would receive a form of clinical management known to be inferior to another. It was thought that perhaps the use of placental grading might be a promising development that could lead to clinical management improving outcome. It was also possible that the clinical action taken on the basis of placental grade would have no beneficial outcome or might cause more harm than good.

Members of the NPEU thought that this method of research was the most intellectually honest admission; that is, since the best approach was not known, the most ethical course of action was to find out which of the two policies was better. In their view, there was no question that this approach was the one most likely to lead to the most appropriate management for women pregnant after the completion of the trial.

The protocol was submitted to the ethics committee for their consideration. In the Peterborough District, this committee is composed of members of the Medical Executive Council plus a lay member who is a solicitor. They examine the protocols submitted for proposed research and discuss the ethical and legal problems that might ensue. All research programmes within the district must be passed by this committee.

When I submitted my protocol, it was referred on two occasions. Some members did not agree under any circumstances that a randomized controlled trial could be used in this way involving women who were pregnant. They came to me personally to explain their views in this respect. The director of the NPEU discussed the problems with the committee and one of the obstetricians was co-opted on to the committee so that he could answer any questions. Finally they agreed that the trial should take place provided each woman received an explanation of it in writing and could refuse to enter if she wished. Written consent was not considered necessary, but informed consent was thus obtained.

THE TRIAL

The trial began on 1 October 1983. Each woman attending the clinic that day and thereafter, receiving a scan at 30–32 weeks, entered the trial in the order in which she attended. Over 3,000 consecutive women were entered. The midwife employed as my research assistant gave each woman a letter of explanation and asked if there were any questions. Providing that she had no objections, each woman's name was then entered into the trial register and given a trial number from 1 to 300. The register contained the trial number with the name of the woman and her consultant's name alongside it. This was the only reference linking the trial number to a name. It was used subsequently to enter other details as they occurred, such as date of delivery, gestational age at delivery, the date the data sheet was completed and sent for computer analysis and so on.

Having been entered into the register, women were then randomly allocated to one of two groups. In the first group, placental recording was reported to the obstetricians for all subsequent ultrasound examinations. In the second group, the placenta was graded but the grading was recorded only for the purposes of the study and was not reported in the case notes. Once entered in the study, the women remained in their allocated group for all subsequent scans.

The following procedure was used for the randomization and data recording. A sealed envelope with the same number as the trial number was issued containing a card and placed inside the antenatal clinic case notes. The cards were of postcard size and of two colours: red denoting the concealed group of the trial, and blue denoting the revealed category. They were placed in sealed thick brown envelopes so that the colour and type could not be seen from the outside, even when held to the light. Each card was also numbered with the trial number. The information on the card included:

1. ethnic group
2. number of fetus
3. if gestational age was confirmed in early pregnancy
4. gestational age at entry into the trial
5. placental grading given at each scan

This information was entered by code into the appropriate boxes. A third party, in our case NPEU, prepared the cards to ensure they were completely randomized.

The woman was then scanned as usual. All measurements and details of the scan were reported in the case notes and on the departmental record card as described. In addition, the ultrasonographer would then open the envelope and, if it contained a card denoting the revealed group, record the placental grade in the case notes, departmental record card and on the coloured card. This information was recorded only on the coloured card if it belonged to the concealed group. A coloured sticker was placed on the case notes and departmental record containing the trial number as a means of cross-reference. Any ultrasound scan the woman received following entry into the trial was recorded in the same fashion. As noted, she remained in the same category for all subsequent scans.

Drill Hall Library Medway

Customer ID: JEF100188242

Items that you have checked out

Title: Appraising research into childbirth : an
      interactive workbook
ID: 6580055206
Due: 20 March 2019

Title:
 Linking research and practice in midwifery : a
 guide to evidence-based practice
ID: 6580090435
Due: 20 March 2019

Title: Midwives, research and childbirth
ID: 6581015852
Due: 20 March 2019

Title: Midwives, research and childbirth
ID: 658004512X
Due: 20 March 2019

Title: Principles and practice of research in
      midwifery
ID: 6580040403
Due: 20 March 2019

Total items: 5
Account balance: £0.00
20/02/2019 11:05
Checked out: 5
Overdue: 0
Hold requests: 0
Ready for collection: 0

Thank you for using the SelfCheck System.

Data collection

The data sheet was printed on duplicated paper so that the top copy could be sent to the NPEU for analysis and the bottom copy kept for reference. These data sheets were completed approximately ten days postpartum but not before. Some were completed at a much later date, so that one could be completely accurate about fetal outcome if there was an element of doubt. The top copies were then sent to staff of the NPEU for analysis.

Problems in the conduct of the trial

It was not surprising that problems should arise in the course of undertaking a project of this size. During the course of this study several events occurred that led to the expected numbers in the trial groups to be drastically diminished.

During 1984, there was a sudden scare about the safety of aspects of ultrasound, caused by reports coming from the U.S. This led to discussions at the Royal College of Obstetricians and Gynaecologists and a report was issued containing certain guidelines for the use of ultrasound during pregnancy. As a result, the obstetricians at the hospital decided they wanted to change their policy of routine scanning in the last trimester. However, the report also recommended that randomized trials in the use of ultrasound during pregnancy were to be encouraged. It was eventually decided that the routine scans would continue in the same way until 3000 women had been entered into the register. One consultant, however, continued to agitate for the women in his care to cease having third trimester scans and insisted that the time element laid down in the protocol be adhered to. It did take somewhat longer, due to the fact that I hadn't allowed enough time for the movement of the population. Several women entered in the trial at 30–32 weeks had moved from the district by the time of delivery, but the response to our requests for information needed for the study was poor.

Another major problem encountered was a change of staff within the ultrasound department. The standardization system first described by Grannum and his colleagues was used for ultrasonographic placental assessment. The grading was based on the appearance of the bulk of the placenta rather than the edges. All scans were performed by two experienced midwife ultrasonographers who had a high level of agreement in this grading of placentae. Thus, in a series of 36 women independently assessed by both examiners, there was agreement in all but one case (which was graded 0 by one and 1 by the other). The final trial size of 2000 was dictated by the fact that a newly promoted ultrasonographer, who did not have sufficient experience to grade placentae reliably, joined the department. Her inexperience was indicated by a low level of agreement with the experienced ultrasonographers when a series of placentae was assessed independently.

Analysis of trial data

For the purpose of assessing the predictive prospects of the trial, we finally chose to look at a 'window' of the women who were scanned between 34–36 weeks (which, as explained, was the normal routine procedure). They totalled 1468 of the 2000 women in the trial. Several women had delivered before this time and some, although having had a scan at the entry time, did not for various reasons have their second and third trimester scan until 36–38 weeks and so were outside the period we had chosen to study. This is discussed further in the analysis of the results.

The predictive properties of grade 3 placentae appearance at this stage of pregnancy for the five pre-specified measures of outcome were expressed in terms of sensitivity, specificity, predictive values and odds ratio, with 95% confidence limits of the odds ratio calculated using Miettinen's method (1976). The birthweight for gestational age standards used were those of Secher *et al.* (1986).

The main hypothesis tested in the trial was that knowledge of the placental grade would lead to clinical action that reduced the measures of mortality and morbidity specified. If the true prevalence of this combination of measures of adverse outcome was 8%, a trial of this size had a 65% chance of a significant result ($\alpha = 0.05$) if the real effect was reduction by a third; the power was 85% if the true reduction was by 40%. The chi square and students' *t* tests were used for the analysis of data.

FINDINGS

Placental grade 3 maturation at 34–36 weeks

Of the 2000 women finally studied, 1468 (73%) were scanned between 34 and 36 weeks gestation. Another 247 (12%) had a single scan at about 32 weeks. The remainder were scanned once before 34 weeks and then for the second time after 36 weeks (usually at 37 weeks).

As shown in Table 5.2, grade 3 placentae at 34–36 weeks, which was observed in 15% of cases, were found to be significantly associated with low maternal age, low parity, low socioeconomic class and caucasian origin. The association with maternal smoking at booking was confirmed: 37% (83) of women with a grade 3 placenta were smokers, compared with 23% (287) of women with grades 0–2 ($p < 0.001$).

As hypothesized, grade 3 placental appearance at 34–36 weeks was associated with an increased risk of meconium staining of the liquor, fetal distress in labour, low Apgar score, low birthweight and perinatal death (see Table 5.3). Although the observed associations are all unlikely to reflect chance alone, none of the associations is strong (the 95% confidence limits shown in Table 5.3 give a range within which the true strength of an association is likely to lie). The sensitivities range from 26% to 57%. The specificity is in all cases near 85%; with the prevalence

Table 5.2 Comparison of socio-demographic characteristics of women with grade 3 placental maturation with women with grades 0–2 at 34–36 weeks

Characteristics	Placental grade				Level of significance
	0–2 (n = 1245)		3 (n = 223)		
	no.	%	no.	%	
Maternal age < 20	134	(11)	48	(22)	<0.001
Nulliparity	601	(48)	149	(67)	<0.001
Social class:					
1 and 2	313	(25)	44	(20)	
3	326	(26)	77	(35)	<0.05
4, 5 and unemployed	580	(47)	99	(44)	
Not known	26	(2)	3	(1)	
Ethnic origin					
non-caucasian	132	(11)	12	(5)	<0.05
Smoker at booking	287	(23)	83	(37)	<0.001

of the adverse outcomes all less than 10%, the implication is that the predictive value of the finding of grade 3 placenta at this gestation is low for all the conditions. Secondary analyses revealed that the associations of grade 3 placental appearance with low birthweight reflects both increased risk of pre-term delivery (odds ratio 1:7; 95% confidence interval 0.9 to 3.0) and increased risk of low birthweight for gestational age (odds ratio 1:3; 95% confidence interval 0.8 to 2.0).

The randomized controlled trial

The 2000 subjects were randomly divided into two equal sized groups. The mean gestational age at entry – and therefore of the first scan – was 31.7 weeks gestation in the revealed group and 31.8 weeks in the concealed group. Randomization also produced comparable groups in other important respects, as shown in Table 5.4.

The clinical management of the trial groups is summarized in Table 5.5. There was little difference between the two groups in the numbers of scans performed after trial entry (mean 1.98 in the revealed group, compared with 1.96 in the concealed group). The main response to the report of early placental maturation appears to have been oestriol estimation. In contrast, the uses of antenatal cardiotocography and admission to hospital differ little between the groups. Despite the fact that induction of labour was less common in the revealed group, delivery tended to

Table 5.3 Predictive properties of grade 3 placental maturation at between 34 and 36 weeks gestation

Characteristics	Grade 0–2 %	Grade 3 %	Prevalence in total %	Sensitivity	Specificity	+pv*	−pv†	Odds ratio	95% CI‡	Level of significance
Meconium-stained liquor	7.5 (93/1245)	14.3 (32/223)	9	26	86	14	93	2.1	1.4–3.2	<0.001
Emergency caesarean section for fetal distress	2.3 (29/1255)	6.2 (14/227)	2.9	33	85	6	98	2.8	1.5–5.1	<0.005
Apgar < 7 at 5 minutes	1.3 (16/1256)	3.1 (7/227)	1.6	30	85	3	99	2.5	1.0–5.9	<0.05
Low birth weight	5.5 (69/1255)	10.6 (24/227)	6.3	26	85	11	95	2.0	1.3–3.3	<0.025
Perinatal death	0.2 (3/1255)	1.8 (4/227)	0.5	57	85	1.8	99.8	7.5	2.1–26.6	<0.005

* + pv = positive predictive value
† − pv = negative predictive value
‡ 95% CI = 95 per cent confidence interval

Table 5.4 Descriptive characteristics of trial groups at entry

Characteristics	Revealed group (n = 1000)	Concealed group (n = 1000)
Maternal age (completed years)		
−mean (SD)	25.8 (5.5)	25.3 (5.1)
Nulliparity	487	509
Social class (%)		
1 and 2	233	241
3	287	258
4 and 5	454	484
Not known	26	17
Ethnic origin − non-caucasian	101	107
Smoker at booking	236	272
Consultant — A	341	350
— B	334	328
— C	325	322
Booking scan	950	960
Gestational age at entry (weeks)		
−mean (SD)	31.7 (1.0)	31.8 (1.0)
Pre-existing medical problems	137	155

occur earlier in this group. This primarily reflected a tendency for spontaneous labour to occur earlier in the revealed group and a high rate of induction in the study population after 41 completed weeks. A caesarean section before labour had started and induction of labour were in fact more common in the revealed group prior to 41 completed weeks. Normal vaginal delivery was slightly more common in the revealed group but this difference was not statistically significant. There was however, a difference in the quality of liquor during labour. Meconium staining and no visible liquor were both more common in the concealed group ($p < 0.025$) and this was only partly explained by the difference between the trial groups in gestational age at delivery.

Neonatal outcome is summarized in Table 5.6. The main hypothesis tested in the trial was based on a combination of measures of adverse outcome. In the revealed group, 71 babies fulfilled one or more of these criteria compared with 83 in the concealed group. This estimated reduction in risk associated with revealed placental grading of 14% was not statistically significant (the 95% confidence interval being a reduction of 38% to an increase of 16%).

The difference observed between the two groups in this respect largely reflected a difference in the number of perinatal deaths in the two groups;

Table 5.5 Clinical management, labour and delivery of trial groups

Characteristics	Revealed group (n = 1000)	Concealed group (n = 1000)
Number of scans after entry:		
1	115	132
2	800	782
3	71	77
4–5	14	9
Oestriol estimation	268	208**
CTG Cardiotocography performed		
number	813	800
mean (SE)	2.34 (0.08)	2.28 (0.08)
Antenatal admissions		
number	312	304
mean stay (SE)	2.52 (0.22)	2.33 (0.19)
Onset of labour:		
spontaneous	717	701
induced	218	237
pre-labour C/S	59	55
not known	6	7
Quality of liquor during labour:		
clear	778	748
meconium-stained	70	101*
blood-stained	73	70
no liquor	16	21
not applicable	52	48
not known	11	12
Gestational age at delivery (weeks)		
mean (SE)	39.09 (0.05)	39.22 (0.05)
< 37	68	61
37–41	925	928
42+	1	4
not known	6	7
Mode of delivery	(n = 1014)	(n = 1011)
normal vaginal	727	709
instrumental	133	143
emergency caesarean	73	81
elective caesarean	62	59
vaginal breech	13	12
not known	6	7

* $p < 0.025$ ** $p < 0.01$

Table 5.6 Neonatal outcome of trial groups

Characteristics	Revealed group (n = 1014)	Concealed group (n = 1011)
Apgar score		
< 4 at one minute	30	29
< 7 at five minutes	12	25*
intubation in delivery ward	20	17
Birthweight (grams)		
mean (SD)	3285 (521)	3305 (555)
< 2500 g	72	75
< 10th centile weight for gestational age	90	88
Admission to special care nursery	48	60
Neonatal seizures	1	2
Antepartum stillbirth	0 (1)†	9 (3)
Early neonatal death	2 (1)	1 (0)
Late neonatal death	0 (0)	0 (0)
Total perinatal deaths	2 (2)	10 (3)*
Baird subgroups of perinatal deaths:		
congenital anomaly	2	3
miscellaneous	1	1
antepartum haemorrhage	0	2
pre-eclampsia	0	2
unexplained > 2500 g	1	3
unexplained < 2500 g	0	2
Perinatal death and/or Apgar <4 at one minute and/or Apgar <7 at five minutes and/or admission to SCBU	71 (2)	83 (3)

* $p < 0.05$
† Figures in parentheses refer to deaths due to lethal malformations.

there were two deaths of normally formed babies in the revealed group compared with 10 in the concealed group. The deaths were subdivided using the Baird system of classification (Baird and Thomson, 1969; Cole *et al.*, 1980). Deaths due to congenital abnormalities could not be prevented by the intervention and for this reason were not included in the combination of major adverse outcomes.

On the other hand, one worry about placental grading is that early maturation might be associated with congenital malformation and thereby lead to inappropriate clinical intervention in these cases. It is therefore reassuring that early grade 3 maturation was observed in only one of the five cases of lethal congenital malformation. One death in both groups has been ascribed to the 'miscellaneous' category and it seems very likely that neither could have been prevented by alternative management in pregnancy or labour.

Details of all the perinatal deaths are given in Table 5.7. The one case of unexplained death in the revealed group had a grade 3 placental appearance at 36 weeks. No special clinical action was taken on the basis of this information. After a spontaneous onset of labour and normal delivery, the baby was born in poor condition (Apgar scores of 1 and 3) and died in the neonatal period. The remaining nine stillbirths were all in the concealed group. There was one fresh stillbirth following an acute placental abruption at 34 weeks. The placenta had been graded '0' at 31 weeks. The second case, ascribed to antepartum haemorrhage, bled on and off for a week prior to delivery of a macerated stillbirth. The placental grades were 2 at 32 weeks and 37 weeks and 3 at 39 weeks. One of the two cases ascribed to pre-eclampsia showed grade 3 appearance as early as 32 weeks but it should be mentioned that other ultrasound parameters, which were reported to the obstetrician responsible, suggested intra-uterine growth retardation; the other case had a grade 2 appearance at 34 weeks. There were three macerated stillbirths with birthweights greater than 2500 grams. One case had grade 3 placental appearance at 36 weeks and one developed the change only after 36 weeks. The third had a grade 1 placental appearance at term and weighed 4430 grams. Retarded placental maturation has been reported in association with gestational diabetes (Grannum and Hobbins, 1982) but unfortunately no glucose tolerance studies were performed in this case. The last two perinatal deaths in the concealed group were classified as unexplained but weighed less than 2500 grammes. One of these cases was placental grade 3 at 35 weeks and was suspected to be growth-retarded on other criteria; the other was also recognized to be growth-retarded and was thought antenatally and at birth to have a congenital abnormality, but this was unconfirmed.

DISCUSSION

The aims of this study were to assess in a total obstetric population the ability of ultrasound placental grading first, to predict subsequent problems, and secondly, to lead to actions that prevent these problems.

For the purpose of assessing the predictive properties of early placental maturation, we chose to concentrate on a 'window' between 34 and 36 weeks because scanning in the third trimester is commonly done at this time, and elective delivery is a much safer option after this time than prior to 34 weeks gestation. Clinical action taken on the basis of a test result may alter the outcome against which the test is being compared and lead to an under- or overestimate of the test's performance. For this reason, the intention had been to restrict the evaluation of the predictive properties of early placental maturation to the group in which the grading results had been withheld from the clinicians. However, the results in the two trial groups in these respects were so similar that we chose to include all cases with scans at this gestational age period to give a larger sample size.

The study has confirmed the association between early placental maturation and problems in labour, poor condition at birth and low birth-weight. Table 5.2 illustrates that if the placenta has matured to grade 3 by 34–36 weeks gestation, there is an association with an estimated increase of between 2 and 8 in the odds of having these conditions. However, none of the sensitivities is high, indicating that only a minority of babies with these conditions (with the possible exception of normally formed stillbirths) will show signs of early placental maturation. Furthermore, the low prevalence of the conditions, coupled with specificities of around 85%, result in low predictive values of positive test results. This means that although the chances of subsequent obstetric problems are apparently more than doubled in association with early placental maturation, only a minority of these cases will actually develop a problem. This suggests that if a placenta is graded at 3 by 36 weeks gestation, it should lead to increased surveillance of the course of that woman's pregnancy and possibly supplementary tests of fetal well-being rather than to more definitive obstetric intervention.

The plausibility of these relationships is strengthened by the finding that early placental maturation is more common in subgroups of pregnant women defined by socio-demographic criteria that are known to be associated with increased risk of poor pregnancy outcome (Table 5.1). The association with early placental maturation and smoking was confirmed. Crawford *et al.* (1985) observed differences between smokers and non-smokers in ultrasound placental texture, as early as the second trimester, that persisted to delivery. In our study, 23% of smokers developed a grade 3 placental appearance by 34–36 weeks gestation, compared with 13% of non-smokers. The nature of the observed relationship with ethnic origin was unexpected: only 8% of non-caucasians (predominantly from Asia) had a grade 3 placental appearance by 34–36 weeks, compared with 16% of caucasians. This was partly but not totally explained by the fact that Asian women almost invariably do not smoke.

The predictive performance of the test – definite associate but poor discrimination – was as expected. It has already been suggested that increased surveillance would be the most appropriate response. Prior to the trial this test was already being used in clinical practice at Peterborough Maternity Unit and no attempt was made to standardize the clinical response in the revealed group of the trial. In fact, the most common response was additional oestriol estimations (Table 5.4).

Randomization generated two trial groups that were comparable in important respects. The concealed group included slightly more women who were young, in their first pregnancy, of low social class, and smokers.

Table 5.7 Details of the perinatal deaths in the trial

Group	Baird class	Gestation (completed weeks)	Birthweight (in grams)	Scan performed (weeks of gestation)	Placental grade	Comments
Revealed	Congenital anomaly	38	1991	32	2	Potter's syndrome
				34	2	Stillbirth (SB)
		39	3130	33	2	Spina bifida Neonatal death (NND)
	Miscellaneous	38	2990	32	0	Good condition at birth.
				35	2	Sudden death on 4th day. NND. Neonatal infection.
	Unexplained (⩾ 2500g)	39	3000	32	2	Poor condition at birth. NND.
				36	3	? birth asphyxia
Concealed	Congenital anomaly	37	2100	32	2	Hydrocephaly and other abnormalities SB
				35	3	
		34	1580	32	0	Hydrocephaly SB
		39	2950	32	1	Spina bifida SB
				33	1	
	Miscellaneous	39	2940	32	0	Good condition at birth.
				36	1	Sudden unexplained death aged 3 days. NND.

Cause	Age	Birthweight (g)	Gestation (weeks)	Parity	Comments
Antepartum haemorrhage	34	2100	31	0	Abruptio placentae at 34 weeks — fresh SB
	39	3133	32	2	Bleeding on and off for the week prior to macerated stillbirth
			37	2	
			39	3	
Pre-eclampsia	32	1050	32	3	Proteinuric hypertension. Small for gestational age (SGA) on U/S — macerated SB
	37	2820	30	1	Proteinuric hypertension — macerated SB
			34	2	
Unexplained (⩾ 2500 g)	38	2800	30	0	Unexplained macerated SB
			36	3	
	39	4430	32	1	Unexplained macerated SB
			37	1	
			40	1	
	39	4250	32	1	Unexplained macerated SB
			37	2	
			38	3	
Unexplained (< 2500 g)	38	1700	32	1	Recognized SGA reduced fetal movement (FM)
			35	3	Unexplained macerated SB
	33	1200	31	1	Thought to be congenital abnormality at birth

These minor imbalances had no important effect on the conclusions drawn from the study. The trial was pragmatic and was superimposed on the ultrasound screen programme already in existence in the hospital. Ninety-six per cent of women recruited to the study had been scanned early in pregnancy and 88% followed the hospital policy and had two or more scans in the third trimester.

The choice of a combination of measures of outcome on which to base the main hypothesis reflected the need for an index frequent enough to allow a reasonable chance of identifying a clinically plausible effect. Furthermore, even using this index, the trial was not statistically very powerful. This is reflected in the fact that the trial's estimated reduction in bad outcome of 14% was not statistically significant. This difference between the groups, however, largely reflected the number of stillbirths (as also did the difference in five-minute Apgar scores). As indicated in Table 5.7, of the (bottom) eight cases in the concealed group which might have been affected by knowledge of the placental grade, three had developed grade 3 placental appearance by 36 weeks, and a further two had grade 3 placenta before term. In the revealed group, the one unexplained death was preceded by grade 3 placental appearance at 36 weeks but apparently no special clinical response was made to this. The observed five-fold risk reduction for normally formed perinatal deaths is certainly an over-estimate of the true effect of this test (95% confidence interval of the relative risk 0.04 to 0.94). Nevertheless, this case review does provide a basis for ascribing some of the observed differences to the availability of the grading information.

The two ultrasonographers who performed all the scans in this study showed near-perfect agreement in their placental grading. Nevertheless, there is no question that the subjective element of the test may result in important inter-observer variation (as has already been described). This may explain the prevalence rates that are different from ours reported from some hospitals (Hill *et al.*, 1983) but not from others (Ashton *et al.*, 1983). Clearly, such variation could prejudice the usefulness of the test. Standardization of the interpretation of the grading system and confirmation of its usefulness in further larger randomized trials is important before the introduction of this test into clinical practice.

By confirming the association between early placental maturation and perinatal problems, this study has provided a plausible basis for believing that routine placental grading in the third trimester may be a useful test of fetal well-being. More importantly, its randomized controlled trial element suggests that clinical actions taken when grading results are reported to clinicians may lead to a reduction in the rate of normally formed intra-uterine deaths. These results suggest that placental grading is one of the parameters that should be reported during third trimester ultrasound assessment of fetal well-being.

ACKNOWLEDGEMENTS

I would like to thank the following people for their help: Dr Adrian Grant of the National Perinatal Epidemiology Unit, Oxford, who helped design the trial, nurtured me through it, worked out the statistics, designed the Tables and assisted in writing, and without whose help the project would never have taken place; Jose Irving-Bell and my colleagues at the Peterborough Maternity Unit; Iain Chalmers and his staff at the National Perinatal Epidemiology Unit; Maws Ltd and the Royal College of Midwives for the award of the Maws research scholarship; the Department of Health and Social Security, which supports the NPEU; and the East Anglian Health Authority for funding the project.

REFERENCES

Ashton, S.S., Russo, M.P., Simon, N.V. and Shearer, D.M. (1983) Relationship between grade II placentas and biparietal diameter determinations. *Journal of Ultrasound Medicine, 2,* 127–9.

Baird, D. and Thomson, A.M. (1969) The survey of perinatal deaths reclassified by special clinico-pathological assessment. In Butler, N.R. and Alberman, E.D. (eds), *Perinatal problems,* Livingstone, Edinburgh.

Cole, S.K., Hey, E.N. and Thomson, A.M. (1980) Classifying perinatal death: An obstetric approach. *British Journal of Obstetrics and Gynaecology, 93,* 1204–12.

Crawford, D.C., Fenton, D.W. and Price, W.I. (1985) Ultrasonic characterization of the placenta: is it of clinical value? *Journal of Clinical Ultrasound, 13,* 533–7.

Grannum, P.A., Berkowitz, R.L. and Hobbins, J.C. (1979) The ultrasonic changes in the maturing placenta and their relation to fetal pulmonary maturity. *American Journal of Obstetrics and Gynecology, 133,* 915–22.

Grannum, P.A. and Hobbins, J.C. (1982) The placenta. *Radiologic Clinics of North America, 20,* 353–65.

Hill, L.M., Breckle, R., Ragozzino, M.W., Wolfgram, K.R. and O'Brien, P.C. (1983) Grade 3 Placentation: incidence and neonatal outcome. *Obstetrics and Gynecology, 61,* 728–32.

Ingelfinger, J.A., Mosteller, F., Thibodeau, L.A. and Ware, J.H. (1987) *Biostatistics and Clinical Medicine,* MacMillan, London.

Kazzi, G.M., Gross, T.L., Sokol, R.J. and Kazzi, N.J. (1983) Detection of intrauterine growth retardation: A new use for sonographic placental grading. *American Journal of Obstetrics and Gynecology, 145,* 733–7.

Miettinen, O. (1976) Estimability and estimation in case-referrent studies. *American Journal of Epidemiology, 103* (28), 226–35.

Quinlan, R.W., Cruz, A.L., Buhi, W.C. and Martin, M. (1982a) Changes in placental ultrasonic appearance. I. Incidence of grade III changes in the placenta in correlation to fetal pulmonary maturity. *American Journal of Obstetrics and Gynecology, 144,* 468–70.

Quinlan, R.W., Cruz, A.L., Buhi, W.C. and Martin, M. (1982b) Changes in placental ultrasonic appearance. II. Pathologic significance of grade III placental changes. *American Journal of Obstetrics and Gynecology, 144,* 471–73.

Schwartz, D., Flamart, R. and Lellouch, J. (1980) *Clinical trials.* Academic Press, London.

Secher, N.J., Kern Hansen, P., Lenstrup, C., Pedersen-Bjergaard, L. and Sindberg-Erikson, P. (1986) Birthweight for gestational age charts based on early ultrasound examination of gestational age. *British Journal of Obstetrics and Gynaecology,* *93*, 128–34.

CHAPTER SIX

Midwives and information-giving during labour

Mavis Kirkham

Women's dissatisfaction with the lack of information available to them emerges repeatedly from studies of consumers' views of maternity care (Cartwright, 1979; Oakley, 1980; Garcia, 1982). As a midwife I became increasingly aware of the misfit between midwifery care and many of women's needs and expectations in this respect. I therefore wanted to examine what actually happens during labour with regard to the flow of information. A DHSS Nursing Research Fellowship enabled me to pursue this objective and undertake the study described in this chapter.

METHODS

I wanted to know what actually happens during labour and therefore chose observation as my principal research method. I undertook continuous observations of labours during which I took written notes. It was not possible to write down every word spoken but it was possible to record some conversations verbatim. Judgement had to be used as to what was written down and this developed over the course of the research. In particular, comments made postnatally by mothers and midwives, as well as patterns that began to emerge from the preliminary analysis of the data, guided my subsequent recording and analysis. Even if these labours had been filmed, these decisions would still have had to be taken later, for as Hanson (1958), a philosopher of science, observed, 'People, not their eyes see; cameras and eyeballs are blind.'

I observed 113 labours: 90 of these were in a consultant unit in a teaching hospital in a large northern city, five were home confinements in the same city, and 18 were in a general practitioner (GP) unit in an adjacent rural area (there was no GP unit in the city). These labours were spread throughout the 24 hours of the day and the days of the year. At the start of each period of field-work, I asked the next labouring woman arriving on the ward whether she was willing to participate in the study. As I wished to observe normal interaction during normal labour, I excluded women who did not speak English, those who were doctors, midwives or private patients, and those whose medical or obstetric history made normal labour or delivery unlikely. Once I had started observations, I continued throughout the labour whatever complications ensued.

With one exception, I interviewed postnatally all the women whose labour I had observed to discover how they saw the labour. In the consultant unit I also interviewed 85 women at approximately 36 weeks gestation to gain a picture of their expectations of labour; I was later to observe the labours of nine of these women. After each delivery I briefly interviewed the midwife who conducted the delivery, usually during the examination of the placenta, to discover her perceptions of the labour. At the end of my period of observation in each setting I interviewed day and night midwifery staff about how they saw their work.

Being a woman, a mother and a midwife helped me fit into labour wards. This also helped me gain research access at all levels, from appearing appropriately professional and humble as a midwife at Health Authority Ethical Committees to being seen as 'one of us' by both midwives and women.

Being a midwife also had its problems. As Pearsall (1965) observed of nursing research, 'a nurse is more likely to overlook what is relevant because she no longer sees it'. In this respect, my viewpoint was widened by childbearing women who, during the course of labour and subsequent interview, showed me the importance to them of things I might otherwise have overlooked. Their observations, values and concepts gave me insights that I would not have had as an ordinary working midwife. This ensured, in the manner advocated by Glaser and Strauss (1967), that my analysis was 'grounded' in my data – data that were also the women's experience.

In working with midwives, there were other research problems inherent in my being a midwife too. As a fellow midwife they often assumed I shared their professional knowledge and views and it was therefore difficult to ask some questions. I was usually able to overcome this by stressing that I was doing research, that I was new to research, and thereby emphasizing the 'ignorant' aspect of my role which required things to be explained to me in a way that would not be necessary with another working midwife.

Trying not to act as a midwife and still be useful was difficult. I decided that I would not initiate action as a midwife but that if asked, I would continue a course of action already started if the person taking that action was to be absent for a short period. Thus on several occasions I continued rubbing a woman's back or holding her hand while the midwife who had started this action left the room to call a doctor. There were occasions when I could not observe this rule; when someone started to vomit and I was the only person with her I found something for her to vomit into. Not to do so would have been inexcusable and would have spoilt future rapport with all concerned. Similarly, on occasions when a labouring woman reached out to hold my hand or arm, I held it. I offered to help on the ward when I was not observing a labouring woman and often, after delivery, bedbathed women whose labour I had observed. I stressed, however, that I could take no part in care during labour, and the staff respected this.

Inevitably, my presence affected what I observed. With midwives this initially had the effect of putting them on their best behaviour. I was quite happy with this as I wanted to know what behaviour these midwives saw as 'best'. I discounted the observations of my first few labours where conversation was full of effusive 'pleases', 'thank yous', and 'excuse mes'. I appeared to be rapidly accepted by the midwives and observed them responding to other more immediate pressures than any caused by my presence.

There was always initial unease with new staff, especially as one sister always introduced me with the words, 'You've heard of big brother. Well, this is big sister.' 'Big sister', however, had no power within the hierarchy of their workplace.

The effect of my presence on women in labour was different. It is more difficult to set formal limits to one's part in conversation than in practical activities. This raises dilemmas when the conversation is a subject of study. On many occasions I was asked questions by a woman in labour or by her husband. I would redirect questions to a member of staff if there was one present, but often there was not. Some questions were directed to me when questioning of staff had proved unfruitful. Sometimes it was clear that questions had been saved for me when no one else was in the room, which in itself is of significance. As a researcher, I wanted to be someone women spoke to. I could not reasonably expect such conversation to flow in one direction only but I did want to observe and not interfere with the flow of information. The way staff dealt with womens' questions early in labour, before any questions were addressed to me, however, showed me how they reacted to the women's search for information.

In the face of my dilemma as a researcher I had also to consider the woman's needs and how they affected her and her relationship with me for the rest of the labour. The continuity of my presence, as well as my marginal status in the hospital power structure, affected the way women saw me, and later many thanked me for being there.

I therefore adopted the following tactics when questions were asked of me. If a member of staff was present, I deflected the question towards her. If the answer to the question was not known, I said so. If the answer might be known later, for instance after the next vaginal examination, I said when that might be. Otherwise I answered questions as honestly as I could. If such an answer was very likely to affect her subsequent conduct, for instance, in refusing analgesia, I continued my observations but did not count that labour as part of my study. Often such answers created a relationship of trust with me which allowed the woman to reveal to me much more of her questions, ignorance, expectations, hopes and fears than she felt able to reveal to the staff. I considered that I was there to learn about the labouring woman rather than to teach her to be a 'patient' by acting as a particularly uncommunicative type of midwife. In many

labours I was asked no questions, possibly through lack of time or incli-
nation on the woman's part. My concentration on my notebook may have
put off many questions and excluded some useful information.

My situation meant that I was acutely conscious of the pressures of
myself as the instrument of data collection and processing. Schwartz and
Schwartz (1955) define the method of participant observation as 'a
process of registering, interpreting and recording'. It is therefore crucial
to be aware of the factors influencing one in 'registering' and 'interpreting'; these include both personal factors and what Baldamus (1972)
called 'the problem of theory determined facts'. I therefore strove to keep
my analysis 'grounded' in the experience of those I observed. The practical aspects of this analysis I carried out by hand. During the field work
period I made some analytical comments in the margin of my notes as
well as a separate 'thoughts' file which fed back into the margin of my
field notes at a later stage. But most of the analysis took place after the
end of the field-work. I developed a card index system for labours and
interviews; as categories were refined, these were indexed back to the
time of the events concerned in the field notes.

FINDINGS

The findings described are those from observations undertaken in the
consultant unit, unless otherwise stated.

Information for women

The women I interviewed were very aware of the extent to which coming
into hospital to have a baby is entering the unknown, even when this was
not their first pregnancy. All the women I interviewed, both antenatally
and postnatally, wanted information with which to orientate themselves
and described their ideal midwife as one who volunteered such information. Mrs 56 said: 'If they don't tell you, you don't know where you are.'
I was repeatedly told: 'You need to know', 'To know so you are
prepared', 'You need to know so you are not frightened', 'As long as I
know what's going on, I'm OK'. For many women, information was what
they wanted most of their midwife. Indeed, Mrs 73 described her as
'being there constantly to tell you exactly what's happening — all the
time. To keep asking if you're all right and tell you exactly what she's
going to do next. Nothing else'. The word 'exactly' was used very
frequently in this context.

The women sought to orientate themselves as to time, place and likely
events. They experienced uncertainty at two levels. First, there is the
physiological unknown of a labour, most of which still lies in the future.
Secondly, there is the hospital and its conduct of labour which contains
social, technical and geographical elements that are unknown to the
labouring woman on admission. They therefore sought information on
both these levels.

Some women conceded that 'there are women who don't want to

know', but no one included herself in this category. Many women voiced the same requirement of the midwife when they expressed the need 'not to be fobbed off', for 'honest answers, not the brush-off'. Some women combined information and support in describing their midwife's job as being 'to talk me through it'. Many women, in their wish for information, acknowledged the uncertainties of labour. Mrs 61 described her ideal midwife as being there 'to tell you exactly what's going on and how long she thinks you'll be, even if she's wrong'. Many women stressed how much they wanted information if labour was not progressing normally and emphasized their need to prepare themselves for what might happen. 'You need to know if things aren't all right. A full explanation. I felt very tense when all the staff were just watching the monitor in silence' (Mrs 87). 'I'd rather know than just look at their faces' (Mrs 49). Mrs 20 expressed these feelings: 'I was at a bit of a loss. Then she said, "If that head doesn't turn, you'll need forceps." I was really glad she said that. I was prepared.' All the women I interviewed wanted to be 'prepared' in this sense.

Patients in other hospital settings gain information from their peers (Roth, 1963). The women I observed laboured in single rooms, rarely saw another labouring woman and therefore, in this respect as in many others, were particularly dependent upon the staff. The staff were important to these women and they in turn were considerate towards the staff. In order to be considerate they had first to learn the values of the staff. The labouring women therefore showed respect for expertise and learnt the priorities of the staff from their actions and the cues they gave.

The admission procedure was observed to be in this sense highly educative for the woman (Kirkham, 1983a) – it marked her admission to the role of 'patient'. The admission form-filling usually started with 'When did your contractions become regular?' Answers to this were often lengthy descriptions of the circumstances and sensations of early labour. The form required a short answer and the midwife usually filled it in with a brief remark such as 'I'll put 4.30'. After that, the woman's replies typically became much shorter. Similarly, if after examining the woman, the midwife told her something of her findings, the woman was likely to ask a question to put this information into context for herself. If she was told nothing, she usually felt she should not ask. The women I observed were very eager to please and do the 'right thing', but their need for information remained. Labouring women used various tactics to put staff at ease and gain information (Kirkham, 1983b). The more successful tactics either emphasized the 'patient's' acceptance of her humble role, for example self-denigration, or were completely passive, for example, eavesdropping or watching and drawing conclusions.

Information-giving by midwives

The importance of giving information was stressed by most of the midwives I interviewed. Their words echoed those the women used in describing their desire for information and showed considerable uniformity and perceptiveness. 'Explain', 'Explain everything you do', 'Don't leave her in the dark', 'Keep them informed', 'Explain the doctor's action', 'Say what you're going to do before you do it', 'Give information to allay fear', 'Talk her through', 'Give information and confidence', and 'Don't fob her off'. These things were said to me repeatedly both as what the midwives felt were important aspects of their work and what they felt women wanted of them. In this context many of them went on to stress that 'everyone is different', so it is important to 'explain at her level'.

I saw information being given by midwives to labouring women, results of examinations carefully explained, and women told what to expect for the rest of their labour. But there was little consistency in the giving of information and much that was not given. At first I thought that this was linked to the nature of the information but this was not so. Much good news was not given, for instance, early vaginal examinations that showed considerable progress already, or low blood pressure in a woman who had reason to fear it might be high. On the other hand, possible abnormalities were occasionally discussed with the woman well before doctors took decisions on them. One of my objectives therefore was to look at the circumstances in which information was given and the manner in which it was given. Various categories were developed from the data in this respect and in the rest of this chapter each is discussed in turn.

Social class, labelling of patients, and the order of the ward

The information given to women and the way they were treated by midwives could to a large extent be seen as a response to the social class of the woman and the tactics used by her and her partner to put staff at their ease. Women of higher social class (defined according to the Registrar General's classification, while acknowledging its shortcomings as identified by Oakley and Oakley, 1979) gained more information from midwives both in answer to their questions and as information offered by midwives unasked. A student midwife said to Mrs 13 (a librarian married to a company director, a former city councillor), 'I assess my patients by their intelligence and see what they will understand. Like you can see that monitor's not working.' (Several women of lower social class in that situation thought the baby's heart had stopped but did not like to ask about it.) 'Patients' of lower social class or less 'intelligence' (in the words of the student midwife quoted above) did not receive more information to balance their lack of it, although my interviews with them indicated that this was what they wanted. They were given sparse information apparently because they were felt to be less likely to understand. Staff seemed to find such women less predictable and trustworthy within the setting of the ward. The emotional order of this setting was a source of security that staff appeared not to want disturbed. They were therefore unlikely to entrust women with information unless the women could in some way set staff at ease and establish themselves as trustworthy in their eyes.

Women of social classes 1 and 2 seemed able to achieve this by their general manner. Staff accepted that they were skilled at seeking information and did not feel them to be disruptive. Women of lower social class either sought information by humble or passive techniques (see Kirkham, 1983b) or in a manner that staff found threatening. For example:

> Labour 82 (teacher married to lecturer):
> Sister's postnatal comment: 'Nice, she was very in control, very sensible.' Throughout the labour Sister told Mrs 82 what to expect next, thus enabling her to feel in control.

> Labour 72 (credit controller married to transport manager):
> Staff midwife's postnatal comment: 'Nice relaxed lady. I think she enjoyed it. That's why I stayed' ($1^{1}/_{2}$ hours after she was due off duty). Mrs 72 repeatedly called herself 'a baby' and used similar terms of self-denigration. Her husband was very skilled at joking and there was laughter throughout the labour. The staff midwife explained the course of labour and the result of each vaginal examination to Mrs 72.

> In contrast, labour 7 (wife unemployed, husband machinist):
> Student midwife's postnatal comment: 'Not doing it properly. This woman wants everything by the book. I was a bit put out by so many questions. I wonder how she'll be with a baby if it doesn't go by the book.' The sister who had supervised the delivery nodded in agreement. Mrs 7 asked frequent questions to find out 'what usually happens' and made a number of enquiries starting 'what if ...' to which sister replied, 'We'll just see what happens.' Very little information was given and remarks seeking information were deflected. For example, Mrs 7: 'I like to know what's happening.' Student midwife: 'You'll be an expert next' (end of conversation).

Staff seemed to find Mrs 7's explicit and unskilled search for information a threat to their composure and the order of the ward. She was not a 'nice lady' in the sense that Mrs 82 and Mrs 72 were, though all three of them were seeking the same information with which to orientate themselves. The staff felt Mrs 82 and Mrs 72 to be trustworthy and to pose no threat to their equilibrium. Despite the midwives' stated desire to give information and their awareness of women's information needs, the need to maintain what Glaser and Strauss (1967) have called the 'sentimental order' of the ward was of overriding importance. This order is defined as 'the intangible but very real patterning of mood and sentiment that characteristically exists on each ward', and seemed to be a crucial source of staff's security which they did not wish to see threatened. As Rosenthal *et al.* (1980) observed of nurses and patients, 'information represents power in the struggle for control and is thus a pivotal question in the study of negotiated order'. The labelling of patients as 'nice' or 'trying to be an expert' and the humble tactics most women used in their attempts to learn made control easier for the midwife. This control included that exercised by those senior to the midwife in the hospital hierarchy. Other factors that affected the midwife in giving information were therefore found in the situation in which they worked rather than in the character-istics of particular women.

The inhibiting effect of senior staff

This was especially clear when these staff were actually present in the room. Midwives appeared less likely to give information to labouring women if other staff were present, particularly if they were senior to them. I repeatedly saw student midwives explain the findings of a vaginal examination to the woman immediately after a sister left the room. Similarly, the sister would explain after the doctor left the room. It may have been in some instances that the person who gave the information had been prevented from doing so earlier because she was busy assisting the senior person while he or she was there. But frequently this was not so; it was the actual presence of the senior person that appeared to constrain the giving of information rather than just providing other things for the junior to do. Perhaps there was an understanding that the giving of 'technical' information is the responsibility of the most senior person present. It was always a doctor who told the 'patient' that she would need a caesarean section, and required her to sign a consent form. Otherwise, information was most often given by midwives, usually in the doctor's absence, or it was not given at all.

Sometimes the limited information the midwife gave reflected the constraints on her actions imposed by medical policies. Such constraints apply, as do the policies, even in the doctors' absence. For example, Mrs 84 had just been admitted in early labour. Sister performed a vaginal examination, then sat on the bed with her:

> Sister: You're only in early labour but you'll get going.
> Mrs 84: On my own?
> Sister: What consultant are you under? What day do you come to clinic?
> Mrs 84: Wednesday.
> Sister: You'll probably have a drip up. What we'll do, we'll do a shave and enema.
> Mrs 84: Enema, that might get me going.
> Sister: Yes. Then, with you being Professor Xs, we'll put you in a labour ward and put a clip on baby's head. Then they'll probably put a drip up.
> Sister then went on to explain the procedure.

I think that sister knew that Mrs 84 was worried about having her labour accelerated. But as that lay beyond her control, she did her best to explain by describing the procedure involved rather than the policy. This dilemma extended to a point where, on several occasions, Sisters said to me later, 'You're called upon to explain these things to patients that you really don't agree with.' These dilemmas are real but they form only a very small part of midwives' information-giving.

The constraints imposed upon the giving of information by senior midwifery staff also appeared to apply in their absence. These concerned the priorities that they were assumed to hold. There appeared to be a very widespread feeling among midwives that it was best to 'say nothing to be safe'. Omitting to give information was not seen as bad care, comparable to the omission of more visible forms of care. I did not observe any student midwife being told to give information to women or being criticized for not giving it. (They were, however, criticized for many other shortcomings.) In this sense, the junior staff's assessment of the priorities of their senior colleagues appeared to be accurate. Indeed, it seemed to be considered wiser to omit information as a precaution against saying the wrong thing.

Verbal asepsis

Dealing with women's search for information within these constraints led to the practice which following Kitzinger (1978), is probably best described as 'verbal asepsis'. For example:

Woman in early labour: I don't know about the epidural. What do you think?
Sister: Let's see how it goes.
End of conversation.

Woman: Is there only one sort of injection?
Sister: Don't be thinking six hours ahead or four hours ahead. See how it goes. I say see how it goes.
Changes subject.

Woman: How long?
Sister: Not long.
Woman: How long's that?
Silence.
Normal delivery three minutes later.

Woman: How long does it take?
Sister: Babies come when they're ready.
Changes subject.

These examples illustrate ways in which midwives blocked conversation by bringing it to an end without answering questions or turned the conversation away from the topic about which the woman sought information. In observing much verbal asepsis, the midwives truly practised a 'linguistic non-touch technique' in that they allowed themselves no contact with the woman's worries or concerns. Furthermore, by thus denying the 'patient' information, they denied her the possibility of any decision-making. Control therefore remained in the hands of the staff.

With such examples from their qualified colleagues, the student midwives quickly learnt these blocking techniques. For example:

Woman in early labour: I don't know what to expect.
Student Midwife: You don't with your first.
End of conversation.

Inexperience

Data from my observations and interviews indicated that student and staff midwives were mostly very aware of the limitations of their knowledge and this reduced the information they felt they could or should give. Yet these were the staff who were asked most questions and had most opportunity to convey information. This was probably because they spent most time with the labouring women and because these women, hesitant to approach more senior members of staff, tended to save questions for periods in which they were alone with the juniors.

On the labour ward little action was observed that might have developed the skills of the junior staff in this respect. The student midwives were keen to learn and this, together with their awareness of their inexperience, led them to adopt the priorities of those who were more experienced. They learnt very rapidly the techniques for blocking and controlling conversation and used them particularly in the presence of senior colleagues. They did give information, but it was not a high priority, and tended to be done in short bursts when sister was out of the room. In these circumstances sister could neither check that the information given was correct nor help the student improve her skills in giving it. Thus, in the sense of teaching or help from those with experience, midwives remained inexperienced in this respect long after they qualified.

Routine patter

The overwhelming importance of pleasing senior colleagues was again indicated in the priority hospital midwives gave to routine. Admission routines are a classic example of this (Kirkham, 1983a). Answering questions and giving information was often, though not always, put off until the routine was completed. This was particularly likely if a sister was present while a student admitted a woman. It could be argued that this sequence of events also constituted that woman's introduction to the priorities of the ward.

Individual midwives developed their own routine patter for giving information. This ranged from such sparse comments as 'I'll just examine you now,' to a running commentary on the labour. Yet other midwives tried to give women a considerable amount of information with which to orientate themselves. Such information tended to be compressed into quite large packages. These packages of information often started with 'What we'll do is ...' followed by an account of the usual conduct of labour in that ward in more or less detail. Those midwives who attempted to give information in this setting (where information-giving appeared not to be valued) must have thought it important. But the pressures on the midwives' time led to the information being compressed into dense routine packages. This led to difficulties for the labouring women who were being asked to digest a large amount of information all at once. Although the fact that information had been offered often made women feel able to ask questions later, such questions often concerned information already given in the initial package. It would have been better if that information could have been given in the context of the labour. While routine packages may be easy for the midwife to deliver, they do not leave room for feedback from the labouring woman. Such patter usually concerned procedures, and lacking feedback, described them as the midwife saw them. Points of most concern to an individual woman might therefore be neglected or omitted.

Requests for information on personal worries outside the routine patter (like all requests outside the routine) seemed unlikely to be met. For example:

> Student midwife described in some detail the procedure for inserting an epidural to Mrs 78.
> Mrs 78: With this epidural, if I was to go to the toilet, would I know?
> Student Midwife: Not always.
> Mrs 78: Oh dear. Would I just go?
> No answer.

The student midwife clearly thought the giving of information important, or she would not have described the procedure in such detail. Having done so, she felt that job was done but left Mrs 78 with her question unanswered and therefore very worried.

The pattern of speech used by the midwife appeared to have a great effect upon the labouring woman in allowing or inhibiting choice. Packages of information that start 'What we'll do is ...' suggest that that is the normal practice and if the woman were to disagree, she would upset the smooth running of the ward. No one was observed to object to procedures described in this way. Patterns of speech that suggested a possibility of choice, for example asking the woman's permission to perform a procedure, suggesting options or even describing a planned course of action with a questioning inflection of the voice, led to women asking for clarification and then taking decisions. This was mainly observed in the GP unit and at home confinements.

Reassurance

The Oxford English Dictionary defines reassurance as 'renewal or repeated assurance'. Assurance is 'the act of making safe, secure or certain, to give confidence, to encourage'. The reassurance I heard midwives use was of two types: reassuring the 'patient' and self-reassurance.

Reassuring the 'patient'. When they felt unable to give information, midwives often gave reassurance. For example:

> Labour 71, while the doctors are outside discussing whether the woman should have a caesarean section.
> Mrs 71: Is everything all right?
> Sister: Dr X is having a word with Mr Y because you're not getting on very quick. It's a long time since you had a baby. We have to keep every eventuality in mind. We keep everyone informed. We tell you what's happening.
> Mrs 71: Is the baby all right?
> Sister: The baby's heartbeat is fine. But it doesn't like the stuff in the bottle. We'll see what Mr Y, the consultant has to say. We're very on the ball here. It's a precious baby.

Remarks such as 'you're in the right place' or 'we're very on the ball here' were common in moments of anxiety, often given in response to specific questions. Such remarks convey no information. Often the reassurance consisted of commands to the woman 'not to worry'. For example:

> Labour 9. After a vaginal examination, the sister asks the student midwife to state her findings which she does in considerable technical detail. Sister turns to Mrs 9: All that means is you're getting on a little bit.
> Mrs 9: Is it all right?
> Sister: Fine.
> Mrs 9: I'm a worrier.
> Sister: Don't worry about being a worrier.
> Sister connects up monitor.
> Mrs 9: I'm notoriously sickly.
> Sister: Don't worry.
> Sister and student midwife leave the room.

The sister felt that she had reassured Mrs 9 and this was confirmed for her as the 'patient' did not again raise her worries. Mrs 9 continued to worry about the progress of her labour, her nausea, and whether she could raise these worries without 'being a nuisance'. She later tried to question other staff when the sister was out of the room.

The Oxford English Dictionary further defines 'reassure' as 'restore to confidence, dispel apprehensions'. But the words of reassurance I heard

midwives use more closely resembled a denial of the woman's apprehensions. For example, labour 5:

> Mrs 5: I'm scared.
> Sister: You mustn't be scared.
> Mrs 5 did not speak again and the only word the midwife said was
> 'push' until the baby was delivered eight minutes later.

Sometimes the midwives reassured in a way that led Mrs 11 to observe
postnatally, 'They treat you as though it's none of your business.' For
example:

> Labour 2. Mrs 2 anxiously watches the trace on the fetal heart
> monitor.
> Staff midwife: Don't sit and watch the monitor. We'll worry about
> that. You can read the paper if you want to.
> Mrs 2: No. I'm all right.

Books on nurse–patient communication condemn such techniques.
For example, Hays and Larson (1963) in *Interacting with Patients*
describe such reassurance:

> attempting to dispel the patient's anxiety by implying that there is
> not sufficient reason for it to exist is to completely devalue the
> patient's own feelings.... There is absolutely no justification for
> trying to reassure, unless you are able to document what you say.

However, the midwife's situation in the hierarchy often prevents her from
feeling able to give genuine reassurance. A classic example of this was
shown in labour 83. Fetal blood sampling was taking place. Three doctors
and three midwives were in the room and had been there for some time.
No information had been given to Mrs 83 since a brief description of the
induction procedure one and three-quarter hours previously.

> Mrs 83 (clearly summoning up her courage to speak): What's
> happening down there?
> Nursing officer: They're taking a little bit of blood out. Don't
> worry.
> Mrs 83: Poor thing [i.e. the baby].
> No further information was given to Mrs 83 until the announce-
> ment of an emergency caesarean section one hour and 28 minutes
> later. She was then distraught.

The nursing officer clearly cared about Mrs 83 as shown by the way she
stood by her head, stroked her hair, mopped her brow and told her how
well she was coping. Yet clearly she felt constrained from talking to her in
a way that might help her to prepare herself for the rest of her labour.
The nursing officer (the most senior midwife present) was worried about
the baby, as was everyone in the room, but all she felt able to say to the
mother was 'Don't worry'.

'Reassure the patient' is a ritual phrase that appears in answer to every midwifery examination question. Reassurance is seen as being a good thing and is not analysed further. Of the several techniques that midwives use to avoid the women's search for information and protect themselves against the risk of saying the wrong thing, reassurance is the most sophisticated. Not only does the woman not raise her worries again but having 'reassured the patient' appears to make the midwife feel better. Such reassurance is, not surprisingly, much used in situations that are stressful for the midwife as well as for the labouring woman. But these are just the situations that commonly precede those emergencies for which the labouring women so wanted to be prepared.

There is now considerable literature on the benefits of information-giving before surgery (Janis, 1968; Hayward, 1975). Midwives appear afraid that women might worry, but the psychological literature suggests that the preparatory 'work of worrying' improves the individual's psychological and physiological coping mechanisms (Janis, 1968). If this work is to be done, it must be aided by the midwife beforehand, for, as the doctors in this study repeatedly told me, 'There's not time to waste explaining once an emergency has been declared.'

Self-reassurance. A number of midwives used patterns of speech that appeared to be designed to reassure themselves that the woman in their care was comfortable and that her needs were being met. For example, labour 86:

> Student midwife after insertion of epidural: That's not bad, is it. It's never as bad as you think it is.
> Mrs 86 does not answer.

The phrase 'that's not bad, is it' was often used, usually after uncomfortable procedures. Women rarely replied. A reply deemed by the midwife to be inappropriate could be dealt with by blocking the conversation, for example:

> Sister: We'll put your legs in these horrible stirrups so doctor can examine you and break your waters.... Let your legs flop or it puts a strain on the top of your legs ...
> After vaginal examination:
> Mrs 18: It's aching.
> Sister: That's pregnancy for you.
> End of conversation.

Procedures were often justified as being necessary in order to give information to the woman or add to her comfort:

> Labour 11:
> Staff midwife: We'll do a vaginal examination, then let you know how you are.
> She proceeded to examine Mrs 11.

Labour 86:
Student midwife explains vaginal examination: It's to let you know how you're doing.

Neither Mrs 11 nor Mrs 86 were given any information learnt in the examinations. This happened frequently and appeared to be a means by which the midwife reassured herself before causing the woman the discomfort of a vaginal examination. These examinations could, of course, have provided much wanted information if the midwife had explained her findings.

Some procedures were justified as being of immediate help to the labouring woman even if the midwife's clinical experience belied this:

Labour 4 immediately before artificial rupture of membranes:
Sister: You'll probably feel more comfortable when your waters have gone.
However, Mrs 4 found the next few contractions very distressing in common with the vast majority of women experiencing artificial rupture of membranes in the first stage of labour.
Labour 7:
Student midwife: You need the drip because you'd be sick if you drank.
Mrs 7 experienced repeated vomiting and retching after the drip was inserted as well as discomfort from the drip site and extreme thirst throughout the labour.

Such justification of procedures appeared to fulfil the midwife's needs rather than those of the labouring woman. When inflicting discomfort upon a woman, the midwife appeared to need to reassure herself that in so doing she was in fact helping her. Or perhaps she felt unable to give or justify the actual reason for the procedure. Doctors made similar statements of justification.

Sometimes midwives appeared to gain similar self-reassurance from speaking for a patient even when she was able to speak for herself. For example, labour B6 (GP unit):

Sister A: Do you want a little drink?
Sister B: I think she should. She's very dry ...
Sister A gets water. Mrs B6 drinks.
Sister B: That's better.

Contrasting settings and the effect on information flow

In the consultant unit, the care given during labour reflected the highly medicalized nature of the setting. The 'patient' was controlled, admitted, processed, delivered and then wheeled out of the ward. Rules and routines for processing 'patients', even routines for making them comfortable, emphasized their role as passive work objects. All labouring women were connected to electronic fetal heart monitors and were required to stay in bed and keep still. If they appeared likely to behave inappropriately, particularly if they were very frightened, epidural analgesia was strongly recommended and 'patients' usually accepted it. Thus complete pain relief was achieved and though fear might remain, the action of staff prevented it being expressed.

If the 'patient' can be seen as a work object in the consultant unit, then the midwife can be seen as the shop floor worker. She does most of the work in processing the work object but the nature of the work is controlled elsewhere. This is true both of the flow of work and the policies, routines, rituals and individual medical decisions that applied to each labouring woman. The labour ward was the doctors' territory and the midwives were responsible for maintaining the appropriate order of that territory. It can be argued that in a setting controlled in this way, their actions in blocking the women's search for information and preventing possibilities for 'patient' choice were the logical action of women called upon to manage such a setting. Only 'patients' who could prove themselves trustworthy or humble, that is, unlikely to be disruptive, were offered information which, if offered to others, might lead to inappropriate patient actions, and thus threaten the smooth flow of work through the ward.

The GP unit was, despite its name, the midwives' territory. The absence of medical staff changed the roles of all concerned. In the consultant unit it appeared that the main person the midwife had to please was the doctor, as the unit was his territory. The GP unit had no medical staff of its own; GPs came only when called and then only attended their own 'patients'. It was the midwife herself who defined the limits of her own role by deciding at what point to call a GP and only the midwives attended all the GP unit's 'patients'.

The GP unit 'patient' could not be completely passive as she lacked the anaesthetic service which brought about that passivity in the consultant unit. In a much more active sense than in the consultant unit, the GP unit 'patient' had to cope with her labour and co-operate with her midwife. Similarly, the midwife had to help her cope and to co-operate for she depended upon that co-operation as she lacked the hospital's array of anaesthetic reinforcements.

The data indicated that women were given more information with which to orientate themselves to their labour in the GP unit. They were also more likely to ask questions and have them answered. All staff were experienced and there were no senior staff to inhibit their information-giving. When a GP unit sister was with a labouring woman, she was likely to give that woman much more of her attention than was possible in situations where she also had to attend to machines, students and doctors. In turn, the women appeared to perceive these midwives as available for questioning. Women in the GP unit were not attached to monitoring equipment or intravenous infusions, and were therefore free to move as appropriate to their own comfort. They were offered back massage, drinks, and advice on breathing and relaxation, and this increased their contact with staff to a level at which they were making choices in order to cope with their own labour. Some of the GP unit midwives' words as well as actions increased labouring women's feelings of being able to make choices. For example:

Sister to Mrs B2: Do you want something for the pain?
You know best.

Turning now to home confinements, the labouring woman's home was her territory and the midwife's role there was that of an honoured guest. The flow of information as far as I could tell was what was normal in that home. The midwife had neither colleagues nor an 'off-stage' area of her own, and her conversation with labouring women was often colleague-like. In the home confinements the women in labour took more clinical decisions (for example, when to have membranes ruptured) than midwives did in most consultant unit labours, and the midwives provided the information and co-operation that enabled the labouring women to make such decisions.

The actions of all the midwives I observed appeared logical within their setting. The flow of information was very much dependent upon the power structure of the setting. In the vast majority of cases, the women I observed during labour 'waited on' the power holders – the men. This was true of women who, while in labour, put considerable energy into 'looking after' their husband as well as 'not being a nuisance' to doctors and midwives. I observed no female doctors. The midwives 'waited on' the doctors in the ward in a general pattern of 'dancing attendance' whose choreography I recorded (Kirkham, 1987). Such actions by all concerned inevitably reinforced the situation which led to them.

On a few occasions (only one of which was in the consultant unit), I observed midwives, 'waiting on' the actual process of birth. They gave their whole attention to the labouring woman; their knowledge and skill was a resource to be called upon as appropriate, not a routine to be imposed. They took their cues from the woman in labour, whereas for the vast majority of women whose labours I observed, the cues they gave and indeed their specific requests, if outside the routine, were ignored. Those who waited on the labour really listened to the woman in labour. While such listening is recommended to midwives (Crowe, 1981), I rarely saw it practised because in the consultant unit the midwife's primary responsibility appeared to be listening to and waiting on the doctor.

It appeared from my observations that this 'waiting on' the process of birth gave immense satisfaction to midwife and mother. It only occurred where the midwife did not have to attend to other women or other professional groups, although I did see it occur in the presence of a GP who also waited on the labour and where there were no mutual expectations between him and the midwife concerning the doctor's status. It did not always occur in the absence of other claims on the midwife's attention, for it appeared that midwives waited on what they trusted, and this in turn was largely determined by the setting in which they worked.

The midwives who waited on the process of birth had gained knowledge and confidence which they conveyed to the women in their care. They learnt from those they cared for, were trusted by them, and worked in partnership with them as respected equals. These were the only occasions in my observations that I saw people working together as equals. The consultant unit 'patients' were, in the vast majority of cases, worked upon. Student midwives did not gain experience in the GP unit; therefore they did not observe and could not acquire the knowledge and skills of those midwives who wait on the process of birth. Because of curren facilities for the provision of maternity services in the UK, the number of confinements taking place in GP units is small. As the midwives working in these units are among the few people in this country who now see normal labour, the opportunities for passing on these skills and knowledge are few. We are therefore in danger of losing these and consequently deskilling the practice of midwifery.

Nevertheless, most labours now take place in consultant units and are managed in accordance with the conventional practices of such units. Midwives learn from what is possible in their work setting and consultant units are the setting of most midwifery education in this country. It is therefore worth looking in more detail at midwives' dilemmas in these units to see how information flow might be improved in any setting.

Language

Language structures our experience in many ways. It provides structure and gives meaning to our perceptions while limiting our thinking to ideas and concepts which that language can express. As the linguist Sapir said in 1928, 'Language is a guide to social reality.... Human beings ... are very much at the mercy of the particular language which has become the medium of expression for their society.' The language I heard on the labour ward was English. Like any other language, English has values built into its evolved structure and usage. In a review of the linguistic literature, Spender (1980) concluded: 'English is biased in favour of the male in both syntax and semantics.' At this very basic level, therefore, the women I observed were using a language tailored in many ways to needs very different from their own.

In addition, the midwives I observed lacked a language appropriate to midwifery. This was clear from my observations and interviews with midwives and students as well as discussion with their tutors and reading their textbooks. The language in which they were taught and the language of the labour ward was the language of the medical profession. This is a language to describe the measurable progress, or otherwise, of a labour. It does not conceptualize the experience of those involved.

Midwives lacked terms to describe the women's experiences. For instance, the 'transition' between the first and second stage of labour, well-described in books written for pregnant women (e.g. Loader, 1980), does not appear in medical or midwifery texts in which stages of labour apply only to physical states of the cervix and the expulsion of the contents of the uterus. Nevertheless, a few observant midwives noticed landmarks in labour as experienced by women. For example:

After labour 63:
Staff midwife: She screamed just before she [i.e. her cervix] was fully [dilated]. I've noticed other people do that.

But lacking the concept of 'transition', she was unable to prepare labouring women for it or to develop specific skills to help women through this uniquely disheartening but brief stage in labour. Indeed, I observed several midwives seek epidural analgesia for women who became distressed and disheartened at this point though by the time the epidural was inserted, the delivery was imminent. These women therefore experienced the additional discomfort surrounding the epidural insertion.

Similarly, I observed a lack of concepts to describe specific midwifery skills. This was true of practical skills and communication skills. Some midwives developed their own techniques in conveying information, such as keeping women informed with a choice of words that conveyed where choice might be possible. This was greatly appreciated but these techniques were not passed on.

Thus, a circle is created. Medical language does not acknowledge midwifery skills or the interaction between these skills and the progress of labour. Therefore, no language has been developed concerning these skills. Although student midwives spend much of their training working with experienced midwives, the experience they must gain is codified in the language of the medical profession and the habits they acquire are appropriate to the power structure of their setting. Without relevant language and concepts, midwifery skills such as information-giving cannot be consciously improved, nor can they be shared, assessed or taught.

To be assessed, these skills would have to be viewed against the background of women's perceptions and experience, as obstetrics does not cover this field. But midwifery adopts only the doctors' yardstick. The childbearing women is the only person involved in her care who has no hand in student midwives' assessments. So, in the strict sense of gaining her qualification, she is the person the student midwife least needs to please.

The power system of the hospital, which originally brought this situation about, creates many self-reinforcing ironies. The 'patient's' politeness and eagerness to please allow the midwives' lack of concepts concerning their needs to pass unchallenged. The midwives, unable to acknowledge and answer women's search for information, take refuge in 'caring' ploys such as 'reassurance' as well as apparently less caring ways of blocking conversation and ensuring that the women remain passive and do not voice their concerns. Thus the language and politeness of the labour ward allows a linguistic semblance of caring and concern while ignoring the needs unmet by the system.

There are thus clear parallels between midwives and those they care for in their lack of an appropriate language. Both are required to speak a language foreign to their needs and concerns. Furthermore, labouring women use techniques with midwives that midwives use with doctors to obtain the information that they need to behave in the way expected of them. Such humility is tragic since by its nature it is not efficient as a way of gaining information and it means that midwives do not achieve their stated priorities in the care they give.

Lacking wider concepts, both labouring women and their midwives could only see as possible what appeared permissible in their setting. In the consultant unit, the permissible was what the doctors expressly permitted or what midwives were seen to do. In that setting, the giving of information was an illicit activity performed when the doctor or senior midwife left the room. Lacking concepts or other models from the class-room, student midwives could only learn from the role models of those who supported the status quo.

Why do midwives lack such concepts? At a professional level it could be due to lack of research and theoretical development within midwifery. But at a more personal level, the midwives in the consultant unit did not even draw upon their own personal experience though many of them were mothers. The midwives who drew on their own experiences and those of women for whom they had cared in labour were those whose work setting allowed them sufficient autonomy to use and develop what they had learnt by experience. These were also the midwives who allowed and encouraged feedback from women. Indeed, in their work setting (home or GP unit) they needed to develop these skills. In the consultant unit, it can be said that the midwives' failure to work towards such concepts and skills reflected their powerlessness there. The midwives there experienced what Seligman (1975) described as 'learned helpless-ness' as a consequence of lack of control in their work situation. While this may be a key part of the learning of student midwives and student nurses in large hospitals, it is not conducive to concept or theory-building.

CONCLUSION

I believe that an awareness of our linguistic habits and the parallels between mothers and midwives in their search for information is a first step to improving our practice. Beyond this there is much that needs to be done in midwifery research and the subsequent development of midwifery concepts and theory. There is little time left to do this, for the majority of midwives are now vastly limited in their practice by the nature of their setting. But midwifery researchers drawing upon the knowledge of those midwives who still retain a degree of autonomy in their practice could feed much of value into midwifery education, as well as raising our consciousness by showing us the nature of our own practice.

To work in this direction to improve our practice as midwives, we need to feel support. I feel that logically this can come from those with whom we have most in common. I have tried to show the immense, sad, common ground between midwives and the women in their care. Midwifery could, I feel, re-establish its autonomy as a result of developing its body of knowledge and skill. This could be done in alliance with women who are developing a considerable body of knowledge of childbirth from the viewpoints of those experiencing it and from such disciplines as medical sociology. Such developments would not threaten the life-saving scientific progress enshrined in our hospitals but would enable the midwife to 'dissect the fat from the muscle in the imputed skill of the professional service worker and to determine the consequences of each for what is done to the client, with what price' (Freidson, 1970).

Can we work towards a situation where the midwife is 'with woman', not just geographically and in her awareness of the woman's needs, but also in her words and actions?

REFERENCES

Baldamus, W. (1972) The role of discoveries in social science. In Shanin, T. (ed.), *The rules of the game*, Tavistock, London.

Cartwright, A. (1979) *The dignity of labour.* Tavistock, London.

Crowe, V. (1981) The midwife and the family. *Nursing* (July), 1171–3.

Freidson, E. (1970) *Professional dominance: The social structure of medical care.* Aldine, Chicago.

Garcia, J. (1982) Women's views of antenatal care in Erkin, M. and Chalmers, I. (eds), *Effectiveness and Satisfaction in Antenatal Care.* William Heinemann Medical Books Ltd, London.

Glaser, B. and Strauss, A.L. (1967) *The discovery of grounded theory.* Aldine, Chicago.

Glaser, B. and Strauss, A.L. (1968) *Time for dying.* Aldine, Chicago.

Hanson, N.R. (1958) *Patterns of discovery.* Cambridge University Press, Cambridge.

Hays, J. and Larson, K.H. (1963) *Interacting with patients.* Macmillan, New York.

Hayward, J. (1975) *Information – A prescription against pain.* Royal College of Nursing, London.

Janis, I.L. (1968) When fear is healthy. *Psychology Today, 1,* 46–49; 60–61.

Kirkham, M.J. (1983a) Admission in labour: Teaching the patient to be patient? *Midwives Chronicle* (February), 44–45.

Kirkham, M.J. (1983b) Labouring in the dark: Limitations on the giving of information to enable patients to orientate themselves to the likely events and timescale of labour. In Wilson-Barnett, J. (ed.), *Nursing research: Ten studies in patient care,* John Wiley, Chichester.

Kirkham, M.J. (1987) Basic supportive care in labour: Interaction with and around labouring women. Unpublished PhD thesis, Manchester University, Faculty of Medicine.

Kitzinger, S. (1978) Pain in childbirth. *Journal of Medical Ethics, 4* (January), 119–21.

Loader, A. (1980) *Pregnancy and parenthood.* Oxford University Press, Oxford.

Oakley, A. (1980) *Women confined: Towards a sociology of childbirth.* Martin Robertson, Oxford.

Oakley, A. (1981) Interviewing women: A contradiction in terms. In Roberts, H. (ed.), *Doing feminist research,* Routledge and Kegan Paul, London.

Oakley, A. and Oakley, R. (1979) Sexism in official statistics. In Irvine, J., Miles, I. and Evans, J. (eds), *Demystifying statistics,* Pluto Press, London.

Pearsall, M. (1965) Participant observation as role and method in behavioural research. *Nursing Research, 14* (1), 37–42.

Pratt, L., Seligman, A. and Reader, G. (1957) Physicians' views of the level of medical information among patients. *American Journal of Public Health, 47,* 1277–83.

Rosenthal, C.J., Marshall, V.W., MacPherson, A.S. and French, S.E. (1980) *Nurses, patients and families.* Croom Helm, London.

Roth, J.A. (1963) *Timetables: Structuring the passage of time in hospital treatment and other careers.* Bobbs Merrill, New York.

Sapir, E. (1928) *Culture, language and personality* (1966 edn). Mandelbaum, D.G. (ed.), University of California Press, Berkeley, Calif.

Schwartz, M.S. and Schwartz, C.G (1955) Problems in participant observation. *American Journal of Sociology, 60,* 343–53.

Seligman, M.E.P. (1975) *Helplessness: On depression, development and death.* Freedman, San Francisco.

Spender, D. (1980) *Man-Made language.* Routledge and Kegan Paul, London.

CHAPTER SEVEN

Is anyone out there still giving enemas?

Sheila Drayton and Colin Rees

Many midwives may feel that research is an activity planned and carried out by experts far removed from the day-to-day reality of midwifery care. In many instances, however, midwifery research has been initiated by an individual midwife who feels that certain procedures are unnecessary, for example, Romney's 1980 study of routine perineal shaving. Others have used research to investigate their beliefs that the quality of midwifery care could be improved through changes in midwifery practice (Kirkham, 1983 and Chapter 6 in this volume; Flint, 1986; Ball, 1987 and Chapter 8 in this volume). Not all these midwives had formal research training, but they all shared a determination to improve care through research and sought the expertise and support of others where necessary.

BACKGROUND TO THE STUDY

The motivation behind the study described in this chapter was the desire to replicate an earlier study on the use of enemas in labour (Romney and Gordon, 1981) to ascertain whether their findings could be validated. The first author also wanted to explore women's perceptions of having an enema and for this needed the expertise of a sociologist, who became her co-researcher.

The use of enemas in labour was questioned by Romney and Gordon in 1981. In their study, the degree of soiling, the length of labour, and the rates of infection were measured in a total of 274 women who were divided into two groups. Women in one group received an enema while women in the other group did not. They found no significant difference between the two groups in the degree of faecal contamination during the first or second stage of labour. Infection rates were similar and the length of labour did not appear to be reduced by the administration of a preparatory enema.

These findings suggested there was little evidence to support the continuation of a practice that has become a traditional part of care in labour. Despite their work, enemas are still a common feature of care in labour in many maternity units (Garforth and Garcia, 1987).

METHODS

In our study, we examined the claims made by Romney and Gordon (1981) regarding the clinical aspects of enemas and like them, also obtained information on how women themselves felt about enemas. The first aim of the study was to establish the clinical evidence for the policy of the routine use of enemas in labour. To achieve this, the following hypotheses were constructed:

1. that an enema results in a quicker labour by reflexly stimulating uterine action
2. that an enema reduces faecal contamination of the delivery area.
3. that an enema reduces the risk of infection to the woman and baby

The second aim of the study was to establish how women taking part in the trial felt about the use of enemas in labour. The two hypotheses relevant to this part of the study were:

1. women who have an enema dislike them
2. if asked to consider an enema in future, women in both study groups would be inclined to refuse one

The study was designed as a replication of the work of Romney and Gordon (1981). The research design was in two parts. First, an experimental approach was used in the form of a randomized controlled trial to test the clinical evidence for the use of routine enemas. Secondly, a descriptive research approach was used to examine the procedure through the eyes of those involved in events surrounding delivery.

Replication studies

A replication study can be defined as the duplication of research procedures in a second investigation for the purpose of determining if earlier findings can be substantiated (Polit and Hungler, 1983). Despite the advantage of validating previous findings, there is little discussion of the replication study in nursing and midwifery research textbooks. In a review of 16 such texts, Connelly (1986) found only two that discussed the topic of replication in any depth. Yet as Fox (1982) emphasizes, they can make a substantial contribution to the body of knowledge on a subject by testing the validity of the findings of an earlier study.

There are a number of forms the replication study can take. Connelly (1986) outlines a range from 'literal' replication, which is as close to the original study as possible, to 'constructive' replication, in which a conscious effort is made to avoid previous sampling and measurement procedures. This last form is an attempt to illustrate that the strength of the findings is not related to the particular sample or the measurement techniques used. Our approach fell into the category of 'approximate' replication, in which there is a change in the sampling procedures but the same measurement methods are applied.

Randomized controlled trials

A possible criticism of the Romney and Gordon study is the non-random nature of the two study groups in the pilot study and the questionable amalgamation of this group with the main study, in which 50 women were admitted to a randomized controlled trial before midwifery resistance to continuing the study brought it to a halt. In the present study, unlike the original, the entire study was conducted as a randomized controlled trial. As Grant (1982) points out, this method is the most appropriate for evaluating alternative approaches to care, as, for example it avoids selection and treatment bias.

Women's views

Increasingly, midwives are recognizing the importance of considering consumer views when deciding on both individualized care and treatment policy. By means of interviews, we explored the views and experiences of enemas through the eyes of the women who took part in the study. This information is as important as the data on the physical effects of the procedure in determining future practice and policy-making in this area.

The study design

The enema used in this study was a low-volume disposable phosphate enema. All women admitted for vaginal delivery with a singleton pregnancy of 37 weeks or more gestation, were eligible for inclusion in the study. Those excluded were women with medical conditions such as diabetes and heart disease, and those with complications of pregnancy such as antepartum haemorrhage and severe pre-eclampsia.

All women who fulfilled the inclusion criteria were told that we were investigating the effects of enemas and asked if they would be prepared to help us. It was explained that if they agreed, they might be in the group receiving an enema or they might be in the group not receiving an enema. Those who agreed to take part were randomly allocated between the enema and no-enema groups. This allocation was carried out separately for primiparae and multiparae. It was planned to recruit 200 women to each arm of the trial.

The midwife who conducted the delivery was asked to record the duration of the first stage and second stage of labour and the level of soiling in each stage. Soiling was said to have occurred if faecal matter was expelled into the delivery area. Romney's and Gordon's findings suggested that an enema does not reduce the incidence of contamination. Our study was designed to replicate their work. Like them, we felt it was important to divide labour into the first and second stage. During the first stage, the woman is passive and soiling is less likely to occur, but in the second stage the woman uses her voluntary muscles to give birth to the baby and faecal matter may be expelled.

The degree of soiling was categorised using the following four point scale:

0 = clean
1 = minimal faecal soiling but no formed stool or appreciable diarrhoea
2 = no more than two formed motions or episodes of diarrhoea
3 = frequent formed or fluid motions

This scale was found to be acceptable and easy to use in the pilot study and was the same as that used by Romney and Gordon. Soiling was recorded separately for the first and second stages of labour. With the help of a research midwife and a microbiologist, all women and babies were monitored for signs of infection. A short structured interview was carried out by a research midwife within 24 hours of delivery to obtain information on the women's views and experiences of enemas.

Pilot study

Following approval by the Nurse Ethics Committee, a pilot study was conducted in order to test the tools of data collection and the method of analysis. The two-week pilot study was carried out in the research site, which helped to prepare staff for the main study. It revealed that the method of randomization produced an imbalance in the proportion of primiparous and multiparous women in the two study groups of 'enema' and 'no-enema'. Few primiparous women were allocated to the enema group, making valid comparisons of length of labour difficult. For this reason, in the main study, those agreeing to take part were first divided by parity and then randomly allocated using numbered sealed envelopes to one of the two groups.

Initially we planned to interview only those women who had received an enema but during the pilot study it became clear that a number of women in the no-enema group were unhappy. They were afraid of soiling during the second stage of labour and in some cases, this inhibited pushing. Therefore it was decided to interview all women to investigate how widespread this fear was.

Main study

The main part of the study covered a ten-week period during which 370 women satisfied the inclusion criteria and progressed to vaginal delivery. Of these, 222 agreed to enter the trial. The numbers declining to enter the study steadily increased over the study period and we discuss this in a later section. Table 7.1 shows the number of women in each arm of the trial.

Table 7.1 Numbers of women in the study groups

Study groups	Primiparae	Multiparae	Total
Enema	50	59	109
No-enema	45	68	113
Total	95	127	222

Source: Compiled by the authors.

FINDINGS AND IMPLICATIONS OF THE STUDY

Duration of labour

Duration of labour was measured in two-hour segments ranging from under 4 to 12 hours plus. The findings were compared for each parity group and, as shown in Table 7.2, there was no significant difference in the length of labour between those who received an enema and those in the no-enema group. These findings, which are similar to those of Romney and Gordon, lead to a rejection of the first hypothesis that an enema reduces length of labour, a commonly expressed belief surrounding the use of enemas.

Soiling in labour

First-stage findings. These first-stage findings, as shown in Table 7.3, demonstrate that 87% of the 222 women in the trial remained clean throughout the first stage of labour. This would seem to indicate that most women are able to control their bowels during the first stage.

Minimal faecal soiling occurred in 8% of women in each group and usually went unnoticed by the woman. Marked faecal soiling (grades 2 and 3) occurred in 6% of those who received an enema and 4% of the no-enema group. The researchers and the midwives noticed that when heavy soiling occurred in the first stage of labour, many women were aware that their bowels were moving and were embarrassed.

The data in Table 7.3 show that there is no statistically significant difference in the incidence of soiling between the two groups when comparing clean with contaminated ($\chi^2 = 0.26$ ns).

Type of soiling. Romney and Gordon's 1981 study suggested that women who are given enemas are more likely to have fluid soiling which can be difficult to control. We therefore decided to quantify the difference in the type of soiling in terms of either formed or fluid faecal material. The faecal material was formed in 11 of the 13 occasions of

Table 7.2 Length of labour

Study groups	Hours in labour														
	< 4		< 6		< 8		< 10		< 12		12+		Not recorded		Total
	no.	%	no.	%	no.	%	no.	%	no.	%	no.	%	no.	%	
Primiparae															
Enema	2	4	12	24	13	26	6	12	7	14	10	20	–	–	50
No-enema	7	16	9	20	13	29	5	11	5	11	5	11	1	2	45
Multiparae															
Enema	28	47	20	34	7	12	1	2	3	5	–	–	–	–	59
No-enema	29	43	20	29	9	13	2	3	5	7	2	3	1	1	68

Source: Compiled by the authors.

soiling in the no-enema group whereas half, 8 out of 15, of the women who had an enema had fluid soiling.

Second-stage findings. During the second stage of labour, only 56% of the group that did not receive an enema remained clean while the corresponding figure was 78% for the enema group, as shown in Table 7.4. In other words, there was a higher incidence of soiling in the no-enema group and the difference was statistically significant (comparison of contamination with no contamination $p < 0.001$). This is in marked contrast to the findings of the previous study (Romney and Gordon, 1981) and may be due to the randomization used in our study.

However, the increase in soiling was mainly in the grade 1 category which was slight and easy to remove, particularly as in 38 of the 43 cases that were recorded, the contamination was formed. The data in Table 7.4 also show that marked contamination was increased in the no-enema group in the second stage of labour but the increase did not reach significance (comparison of contamination level $0 + 1$ v. $2 + 3$).

Table 7.3 Soiling in the first stage of labour

Study groups	Soiling rating								
	Clean		1		2		3		Total
	no.	%	no.	%	no.	%	no.	%	
Enema	94	86	9	8	6	6	–	–	109
No-enema	100	88	9	8	3	3	1	1	113

Source: Compiled by the authors.

Table 7.4 Soiling in the second stage of labour

Study groups	Soiling rating								
	Clean		1		2		3		Total
	no.	%	no.	%	no.	%	no.	%	
Enema	85	78	20	18	3	3	1	1	109
No-enema	63	56	39	35	9	8	2	2	113

Source: Compiled by the authors.
Comparison of soiling with no soiling: $p < 0.001$

From the comments made in the interviews, it became clear that during the second stage of labour many women were unaware of soiling and even repeated soiling went unnoticed.

Types of soiling. We were anxious to quantify the type of soiling in the second stages of labour and therefore we were disappointed to find that this information had not been recorded in 2 of the 24 cases of soiling in the enema group and in 7 of the 50 cases of soiling in the no-enema group. However, the recorded findings were sufficient to show that fluid soiling occurred in 12 (50%) of the enema group and 5 (10%) of the no-enema group. This difference is highly significant ($p < 0.001$).

The results show that if women labour without an enema, most of them will remain clean throughout the first stage. Some 35% will have minimal faecal soiling in the second stage of labour but this is easy to remove, particularly as the faecal matter is usually formed. In most instances, it is unlikely to cause embarrassment to the women and we suggest it is acceptable to most midwives as 'manageable'.

Our study shows that this percentage of soiling can be reduced by the administration of a preparatory enema but that the reduction is bought at the expense of a shift from formed to fluid motions which tend to contaminate more widely and which are more difficult to remove from the delivery area. It might also be possible to reduce this percentage by simply asking women to move their bowels at the onset of labour. We were told by one participant, a Malaysian woman, that this is the custom in her country and we feel that such a simple method should be tried and evaluated.

For those midwives and doctors who find minimal soiling in 35% of women unacceptable, the effectiveness of suppositories could also be investigated. But in our view it is doubtful whether all faecal material would be expelled from the lower bowel and therefore minimal soiling might still occur in the second stage of labour.

Marked faecal soiling in labour remains a problem. It is embarrassing for the women, particularly in the first stage of labour, and it can be difficult to control. Ten per cent of women in this study were affected and this percentage was not significantly reduced by the administration of a small-volume disposable enema. The problem of marked soiling needs further study.

In our view these findings do not support the routine use of enemas in labour but point to the need to assess the state of the bowel of women in early labour and to develop care plans tailored to individual needs.

Infection

Infection was confirmed in 13 babies; 6 were in the enema group and 7 in the no-enema group. One baby in each group had an umbilical infection that could be related to bowel organisms, *E. coli* and *streptococcus faecalis* respectively. None of the women had a perineal wound infection.

Despite a higher incidence of soiling in those women who did not receive an enema, there was no difference in the infection rate. In other words, the third hypothesis that an enema reduces the risk of infection in mother and baby can also be rejected.

The views of the women

In addition to the clinical aspect of the study, we interviewed the women in both groups to establish how they felt about enemas and whether they would accept one in a future delivery. The women were asked if they had expected to receive an enema as part of the normal delivery procedures and the overwhelming majority (88%) said that they had expected one. Only one person said, 'Never heard of them'. How then did those who received an enema feel about the experience and by comparison, how did those who were expecting one but did not receive one, feel about the situation?

Those in the experimental group were asked to describe the experience of having an enema. The comments varied considerably, with some women feeling 'there was nothing to it' while others gave quite graphic descriptions of discomfort and personal upset. The comment from one of this latter group was as follows.

It stung and got awfully painful. I would say it was as bad as contractions. I had very liquid diarrhoea which seemed to go on for ages and then in the middle of all that the contractions got stronger. I wouldn't have minded the contractions but what with the diarrhoea and being in the toilet, it was horrible hell.

Romney and Gordon (1981) similarly quote one woman who feared that she was on the verge of delivery while sitting alone on the toilet.

Table 7.5 shows the range of comments analysed under key headings and divided by parity. As respondents sometimes made a number of comments, the percentages in this table total more than 100%. It is clear that there is a pattern of response by parity. A far larger proportion of primiparous women compared to multiparous women said 'it was not as bad as expected' ($p < 0.005$). This suggests that quite a large number of women undergoing delivery for the first time experienced anticipatory anxiety.

The data in Table 7.5 show that a substantial proportion of women found the experience of having an enema distressing. This underlines the importance of evaluating the efficacy of routine procedures as they may cause physical distress for no proven benefit. Delivery can be a painful and anxious event without adding further discomforts.

Turning to the group who did not receive an enema, they were asked, 'How did you feel when you were told that you would not be receiving an enema?' The replies to this question are shown in Table 7.6.

Table 7.5 How would you describe the experience of having an enema

Descriptions	Total (n = 109)		Primiparae (n = 50)		Multiparae (n = 59)	
	no.	%	no.	%	no.	%
Not as bad as expected nothing to it	47	43	29	58	18	31
Physical description cold, weak, faint	32	29	17	34	15	25
Discomfort uncomfortable/unpleasant	33	30	14	28	19	32
Positive effect cleared me out/helped	14	13	6	12	8	14
Psychologically secure felt safe etc.	8	7	–	–	8	14
Psychological insecurity worried/anxious	4	4	2	4	2	4
Embarrassing	2	2	–	–	2	4
No particular opinion doesn't bother me	5	5	3	6	2	4
Other	5	5	2	4	3	5
Women discharged before interview	6	5	1	2	5	8

Source: Compiled by the authors.

The response made most frequently was 'relieved/delighted' which was stated by just under half of those in this group. Again, there are differences by parity, with a larger proportion of multiparous women falling into this category. Presumably they have a more accurate knowledge of what an enema would mean. Conversely, the primiparous group were more likely than the multiparous group to say they were 'unconcerned' or 'did not mind' (40% compared with 22%). The other responses listed in the table were each made by much smaller proportions of the respondents.

Both those in the enema and no-enema group were asked what their reactions would be on a future occasion if they were offered an enema. In the interview, each respondent was given a card with a number of fixed alternatives and asked to choose the one she felt was closest to the way she might respond. The findings are shown in Table 7.7.

The most frequent response in both groups was 'would not mind one way or the other' with an almost identical proportion in each group

Table 7.6 How did you feel when told you would not be given an enema

Feelings	Total (n = 113)		Primiparae (n = 45)		Multiparae (n = 68)	
	no.	%	no.	%	no.	%
Relieved/delighted	49	43	17	38	32	47
Unconcerned/didn't mind	33	29	18	40	15	22
Apprehensive/anxious/ nervous	8	7	3	7	5	7
Mixed feelings – relieved but anxious in case of accidents	4	4	2	4	2	3
Surprised	2	2	1	2	1	4
Disappointed	2	2	1	2	1	2
Wasn't expecting one/never heard of them	1	1	–	–	1	2
Women discharged before interview	14	12	2	4	12	18

Source: Compiled by the authors.

Table 7.7 Respondents' feelings about a future enema by group

Feelings about a future enema	No-enema group		Enema group	
	no.	%	no.	%
Wouldn't mind one way or other	45	40	47	43
Willingly accept*	14	12	41	38
Accept with some reluctance	26	23	11	10
Strongly object	14	12	4	4
Women discharged before interview	14	12	6	6
Total	113	100	109	100

Source Compiled by the authors.
* $p < 0.01$

answering in this way. The distribution among other alternatives, however, is not the same in the two groups. Those who did not have an enema this time were far less likely to say they would 'willingly accept' but were more likely to accept only with some reluctance or strongly object to one.

These data were then analysed by parity and the results are shown in

Table 7.8. The percentage of respondents choosing the alternative 'willingly accept' suggest that the routine nature of a procedure may play a part in achieving patient compliance. Starting with primiparous women in the no-enema group, who are unlikely to have experienced an enema previously and were not given one on this occasion, only 9% said they would willingly accept a future enema. This figure rises to 15% for multiparous women who may have had a previous enema but did not have one on this occasion. In the enema group, the proportion rises to 32% for primiparae and even further to 42% for multiparous women who have probably had an enema before and also had one on this occasion. This rising trend may well be explained by the role of tradition in achieving compliance, in that if you give someone what they believe is good for them because it is 'accepted practice', they will be willing to have it again. If this is reinforced on a future occasion, then the belief in its importance increases even further, as can be seen in those multiparous women who had an enema this time. On the other hand, if women are put in a similar situation and it is not reinforced, then there is a reduction in compliance as can be seen in the multiparous women who did not have an enema this time. This group may well have questioned whether an enema is really necessary on all occasions.

It is suggested that patient compliance with painful and uncomfortable procedures can be maintained by making them a routine for everyone. Once we provide options for a routine procedure, then people begin to question their relevance in all circumstances. In the case of enemas, the

Table 7.8 Feelings about a future enema by parity

Feelings about a future enema	No-enema group				Enema group			
	Primiparae		Multiparae		Primiparae		Multiparae	
	no.	%	no.	%	no.	%	no.	%
Wouldn't mind one way or other	22	49	23	34	25	50	22	37
Willingly accept	4	9	10	15	16	32	25	42
Accept with some reluctance	10	22	16	24	6	12	5	9
Strongly object	7	16	7	10	2	4	2	3
Women discharged before interview	2	4	12	18	1	2	5	9
Total	45	100	68	100	50	100	59	100

Source: Compiled by the authors.

community served by the maternity unit held the expectation that the procedure would be routinely given and therefore there must be a good reason for it. This view may well have been supported by midwifery staff who have long been familiar with the beliefs surrounding the use of enemas in labour and so feel it is an essential part of 'prepping'. However, once the midwife sees that the consequences of a delivery without a routine enema are not catastrophic, then her belief in the necessity of enemas may diminish.

It might have been anticipated that if soiling took place during labour, then the individual would be more inclined to willingly accept an enema in the future. This was not the case, as only 15% of those who soiled chose this option. This supports the earlier statement that where soiling had taken place, many women were unaware of it.

Women were also asked why they had chosen a particular option in relation to having an enema in the future. The analysis of their comments led to the development of a further theme, the 'good sense' attributed to midwives by those in their care. This was demonstrated by respondents who on the one hand chose the alternative that they would accept a future enema 'with some resistance' but then went on to say, 'I wouldn't object if advised to have one but feel it is really unnecessary'. Another stated, 'if the midwife advised me to have one, then I would take her advice'. Awareness of this acceptance of professional judgement is important as it places a responsibility on the midwife to ensure that there are good grounds for the decision she makes rather than basing activities simply on long-established routines.

DISCUSSION

In this study, an attempt has been made to produce reliable findings through the use of a randomized controlled trial. Three points should be emphasized in relation to the conduct of research. First, the midwife need not undertake such a venture alone. Here, collaboration provided a balance between midwifery skills and research knowledge. A team approach as in this study, providing a combination of midwifery and research skills, has much to commend it. Secondly, there was a conscious decision at the outset that the study would not just focus on physical aspects of care but would also include the views of those on the receiving end of the treatment. This was an important addition as it has indicated the creation of compliance through routine application of certain procedures. The findings clearly show that those who received an enema and were probably expecting one on the basis of previous experience, would be happy to receive one in the future as the professional 'must have a good reason for using it'. This phenomenon of 'they know what they're doing' (Drayton and Rees, 1984) has also been found in other areas of care where the acceptance of the present routine as 'best', if supported by obstetric and midwifery staff, has been demonstrated (Porter and Macintyre, 1984).

Thirdly, problems were encountered in the conduct of the trial itself. In both this study and that of Romney and Gordon (1981), the trial had to be curtailed sooner than planned because some of the midwives ceased to adhere to the trial protocol. They did this because, having observed on an individual basis that women came to no harm if they did not have an enema, they advised them not to enter the trial in case they ended up in the group receiving an enema. The study indicated that involving midwives in locally based research projects may be more effective in encouraging them to accept research findings than from just reading reports of studies carried out by others. None the less, if results of such studies are to be valid and accepted by practitioners elsewhere, it is essential that researchers ensure that all involved are aware of the importance of adhering to the protocol. In relation to the clinical questions surrounding the routine use of enemas, the results of this study support earlier work demonstrating that one of the main beliefs surrounding enemas, namely that they result in quicker labour, cannot be supported by empirical evidence.

Although there is the possibility of a higher incidence of soiling in the delivery area, this is not accompanied by a higher infection rate. In other words, there appears to be little evidence to support the routine use of enemas for all women in labour.

It is likely that soiling can be maintained at an acceptable level by encouraging women to open their bowels themselves during the first stages of labour. In some cases, however, where this does not empty a full or impacted bowel, additional steps may be necessary. From our findings, however, it appears that in such cases a small-volume enema may not always be effective. Further work is necessary to look in more detail at such cases.

We would argue for a more personalized approach to this area of delivery with treatment tailored to the individual's needs. The consequences of a labour without an enema are certainly not catastrophic and their continued routine use cannot be justified. The problem is that enemas have been a part of labour for so long that both staff and women themselves have come to regard them as an essential part of the labour process.

Nevertheless, the views of staff should be amenable to change in the light of all the evidence. In our study, we found that the attitude of women who have been influenced by the midwifery world's longstanding faith in enemas may be more difficult to change. Following our work and that of previous authors, we hope that in the future the answer to the question 'is anyone out there still giving enemas?' will be 'only when the individual case necessitates'.

One frustration for the researcher is the time lag between the publication of findings that have important consequences for practice, and their acceptance by practitioners and their inclusion in education programmes. This has been well-illustrated by Walton (1985) in relation to perineal shaving. Garforth and Garcia (1987) have demonstrated a number of routine practices in admission that have survived despite research evidence that questions their value. In relation to enemas, only 16% of the districts in their study had a policy of no routine bowel preparation. Why should this practice persist? We believe it is the routine nature of preparatory enemas that has largely been responsible for their continued use. Until obstetricians and midwives question their use and replicate studies like the one reported here, many women will continue to undergo a procedure that for some is feared more than delivery itself.

REFERENCES

Ball, J.A. (1987) *Reactions to motherhood – the role of postnatal care.* Cambridge University Press, Cambridge.

Connelly, C.E. (1986) Replication research in nursing. *International Journal of Nursing Studies, 23* (1), 71–77.

Drayton, S. and Rees, C. (1984) 'They know what they're doing'. *Nursing Mirror* (Midwifery Forum), *159* (3), iv–viii.

Flint, C. (1986) The 'know your midwife' scheme. *Midwife, Health Visitor and Community Nurse,* May *22* (5), 168–9.

Fox, D.J. (1982) *Fundamentals in nursing research* (4th edn). Appleton-Century-Crofts, New York.

Garforth, S. and Garcia, J. (1987) Admitting – a weakness or a strength? Routine admission of a woman in labour. *Midwifery, 3* (1), 10–24.

Grant, A. (1982) Evaluating midwifery practice: The role of the randomised controlled trial. In Thomson, A. and Robinson, S. (eds), *Research and the Midwife Conference Proceedings,* Manchester University.

Kirkham, M. (1983) Admission in labour: Teaching the patient to be patient. *Midwives' Chronicle, 120* (February), 44–45.

Polit, D.F. and Hungler, B.P. (1983) Nursing research: Principles and methods (2nd edn). Lippincott, Philadelphia.

Porter, M. and Macintyre, S. (1984) What is must be: A research note on conservative or deferential responses to antenatal care provision. *Social Science and Medicine, 19* (11), 1197–1200.

Romney, M.L. (1980) Pre-delivery shaving: An unjustified assault? *Journal of Obstetrics and Gynaecology, 1,* 33–35.

Romney, M.L. and Gordon, H. (1981) Is your enema really necessary? *British Medical Journal, 282,* 1269–71.

Walton, J.G. (1985) Information and the midwife. *Midwifery, 1* (4), 191–4.

CHAPTER EIGHT

Postnatal care and adjustment to motherhood

Jean A. Ball

INTRODUCTION

The process of adjustment to motherhood is neither simple nor easy. It is marked by physical, psychological and emotional change. During this time the mother recovers from the physiological changes of pregnancy, the trauma of labour and delivery, and learns and develops the skills necessary for the care of her baby. There are also changes in family relationships and social networks as she and her husband undertake the demanding, satisfying, daunting and joyful responsibilities of parenthood. It is not surprising, therefore, to find pregnancy and childbirth listed among major life-events (Holmes and Rahe, 1967), or described as peak developmental experiences by psychologists (Erikson, 1963; Rapoport, Rapoport and Strelitz, 1977; Brown, 1979).

Studies of postnatal depression indicate that 10% of mothers suffer from depression of sufficient severity to warrant psychiatric intervention, while a further 10% experience considerable emotional distress and disturbance for several weeks and months following the birth of a baby (Tod, 1964; Pitt, 1968; Kumar and Robson, 1978; Cox *et al.*, 1982). If we consider that approximately 600,000 babies are born each year in England and Wales, this evidence indicates that the lives of 60,000–120,000 families are currently impoverished by this distressing illness, making postnatal depression or distress one of the major causes of post-natal morbidity. It is surprising, therefore, that until recently little attention has been paid to this situation, and that little information about the processes that underlie adjustment to motherhood is to be found in obstetric and midwifery textbooks.

The research described in this chapter arose from a desire to understand more fully the various factors that influence the emotional response to motherhood, and to examine the degree to which current patterns of postnatal care given by midwives assist or detract from the adjustment process. The concepts of the coping process (Lazarus, 1966) and the role of support systems (Caplan, 1964) were used as the theoretical framework of the study. Lazarus describes the following three interacting components of the way in which individuals respond to change or stress:

antecedent factors, such as personality and previous learning experiences that predispose the response and maintain consistency with the person's normal patterns of behaviour; the immediate emotional and physical response to the situation; and the outcome in terms of behaviour that enables an individual to overcome or come to terms with a particular situation.

The nature of the outcome in terms of coping behaviour will be determined by the factors noted above, and by the quality and degree of the support that an individual has available to assist him during the period of crisis. Anxiety is a potent factor in this process and may be present as an antecedent factor in the form of a stable personality trait, and may also emerge as part of the reaction to stress. In some situations, anxiety will remain as part of the coping behaviour (Lazarus, 1969). Caplan (1969) places great emphasis on the socio-cultural environment and its influence, and considers that an individual experiencing stress is more susceptible to the influence of others during the period of adjustment than at times of normal functioning. For this reason Caplan asserts that the role of the professional or lay helper may be crucial in determining the outcome in terms of speed of adjustment and subsequent emotional health. He lays great emphasis, therefore, on the need for professional care-givers to develop insight and understanding of the pyschological needs of their clients.

Previous research has identified a number of antecedent and con-current factors that make a woman more vulnerable to emotional distress and depression both in the postnatal period and at other times of stress. These illustrate further the concepts of the coping process described by Lazarus and Caplan. These factors may be described as antecedent or predisposing factors, or as stress factors. Antecedent factors include an anxious personality (Tod, 1964; Pitt, 1968; Kumar and Robson, 1978, 1984), and separation from own mother in childhood (Frommer and O'Shea, 1973; Brown and Harris, 1978). The stress factors identified centre particularly on marital tension, especially the lack of a confiding, trusting relationship with the husband or male partner (Tod, 1964; Stott, 1973; Kumar and Robson, 1978, 1984), and social and financial stresses (Nuckolls, Cassell and Kaplan, 1972; Oakley, 1980).

In view of the many factors involved in maternal emotional reactions to childbirth and motherhood, the question upon which the research was based was defined as follows:

> In view of the many internal and external factors that influence maternal response to childbirth and mothering, what effect, if any, do the current patterns of postnatal care given by midwives in the National Health Service have upon the adjustment process?

STUDY DESIGN AND METHODS

It was necessary that the research should be designed in a way that would take note of the factors in the maternal and family situation that were likely to affect the mother's response, in order to distinguish their effects from those that arose from the pattern of postnatal care. Accordingly, two hypotheses were formulated upon which the design was based.

Hypothesis 1: The emotional response of women to the changes which follow the birth of a child will be affected by their personality, and the quality of the support they receive from their personal and social support systems.

Hypothesis 2: The way in which care is given by midwives during the postnatal period will influence the emotional response of women to the changes which follow the birth of a child.

The work was designed as a descriptive and analytic study of the experiences and perceptions of women during the first six weeks of the life of their baby as they adapted to and coped with the demands that the birth of the baby made upon themselves and their family. It was mainly prospective in nature, but contained a retrospective assessment by the mother of the events of her labour, delivery and of the postnatal care she received both in hospital and in the community. The mother's self-assessment of her emotional well-being six weeks after the birth of her baby was defined as the dependent variable. Her satisfaction with motherhood at this time was defined as the secondary dependent variable.

The research instruments to be used, therefore, were designed to allow for an examination of the effects that the many different events and circumstances might have upon the dependent variables, and a firm basis for statistical analysis was incorporated into the design. Further details of the research design and the results can be found in associated work (Ball, 1983, 1987).

Major variables included in the design

Antecedent factors. These data, which were collected during the antenatal interview, include the following:

1. maternal personality was assessed by the use of the Eysenck Personality Inventory (Eysenck and Eysenck, 1968). This had the advantage of being readily administered by a non-psychologist and allowed direct comparison of results with the previous studies by Pitt (1968) and Kumar and Robson (1978).
2. previous history of maternal separation from her own mother during childhood (Frommer and O'Shea, 1973; Brown and Harris, 1978)
3. life crisis events affecting the mother or her immediate family during the year preceding the birth of the baby
4. mother's social class, parity, marital status and family circumstances

Process and events of childbirth and the puerperium. The events of the labour and delivery were obtained from the hospital record. The mother's perception of these events, her recall of her first physical contact with her baby, and the time of the first feed she gave to her baby were obtained during a postnatal interview which took place within 24–48 hours of the birth. The mother's perception of labour and delivery was obtained by discussion and by the completion of a five-point rating scale.

The events of the postnatal period spent in hospital were obtained from the hospital records, by observation of the patterns of care operated on the ward, and by discussion with the midwives concerned. An interview was held in each case with the hospital midwife who arranged for the mother and baby's transfer home, and this took place on the day that the mother was discharged. During the interview the midwife was asked about her perceptions of the mother's needs in feeding and caring for her baby, and of her emotional status during her stay in the ward.

The events of the postnatal period, during which the mother was visited by the community midwifery services, were obtained by a questionnaire sent to the appropriate midwife on the day the mother was discharged to her care, and completed by the midwife on the day that the mother was finally discharged from the maternity services. The questionnaire contained details of the pattern of feeding, degree of family support, mother's emotional reactions, and the time of discharge from community care.

The mother's perceptions of these events, her reactions to the care she received, and her feelings about herself during the time of postnatal care in hospital and in the community was obtained by a retrospective assessment contained in a questionnaire sent to her when the baby was six weeks old.

Measures of outcome. The mother's self-assessment of her emotional well-being, satisfaction with motherhood, and the degree of family support being provided six weeks after the birth of the baby was obtained by use of a second questionnaire. The statements in the questionnaire were based upon the Beck Depression Inventory (Beck *et al.*, 1961), the questionnaire used by Pitt (1968), and the work of Klaus and Kennell (1976, 1982). A further measure of maternal well-being and satisfaction with motherhood was obtained by the use of a scale based upon the Broussard Neonatal Perception Inventory (Broussard and Hartner, 1971).

Structure of the questionnaires

The postnatal perception questionnaires and the emotional well-being and satisfaction with motherhood questionnaire consisted of a series of statements. The mother was asked to indicate which of five structured responses to each statement most nearly reflected her feelings about the particular item. The method was based upon those commonly used in attitude surveys (Oppenheim, 1966; Treece and Treece, 1977) and the five-point scoring scale was based upon methods used by Likert (1932).

The emotional well-being/satisfaction with motherhood questionnaire was made up of 32 statements. The measure of emotional well-being arose from 19 statements based upon the work of Beck *et al.* (1961) and Pitt (1968). These statements concerned the presence or absence of various depressive symptoms ranging from anxiety, depression and irritability, to sleep disturbance and loss of appetite and libido. Seven statements related to satisfaction with motherhood rated the mother's confidence and pleasure in her mothering role and in the developing relationship between mother and baby. The remaining six statements in the questionnaire were concerned with the mother's perception of the support she was receiving from her family and friends.

The statements in the questionnaire were phrased in either negative or positive terms and distributed in such a way as to prevent a response set (Oppenheim, 1966). For example, two statements concerned with mood are shown below:

I feel full of energy these days.
I've felt low in spirits since my baby was born.

To these and every statement the mother indicated one of five responses: Strongly Agree, Agree, Neither Agree nor Disagree, Disagree, Strongly Disagree.

The score system rated the response from one to five in such a way as to give the highest score to the most positive response. Thus, if the answer to 'I feel full of energy' was Strongly Agree, a score of five would be given; but an answer of Disagree would obtain a score of two. On the other hand, a negatively phrased question, such as 'I've felt in low spirits since my baby was born', would receive a score of one if the answer was Strongly Agree, and a score of four if the answer was Disagree. This pattern of negative and positive statements and the scoring pattern described was used in the postnatal care and emotional well-being questionnaires.

The postnatal care in hospital questionnaire consisted of 16 statements, and that concerned with postnatal care in the community contained 14 statements.

Factor analysis of the questionnaires

The scores given by each mother to the statements on the questionnaires were subjected to factor analysis. This is a statistical technique that identifies the way in which scores given to individual questions are linked together because the responses arise from a common source or attitude. The commonality of the responses is shown by the degree of correlation between them (Oppenheim, 1966; Stopher and Meyburg, 1979).

By using this technique it is possible to identify factors that underlie the way the responses are made and, thus, to expand the understanding of the feelings being expressed and to simplify the analysis of the findings by using the factor scores rather than the scores for each individual question. Another advantage of using factor analysis is to reduce the possibility of distortion, because the factors identified arise from the analysis of the mother's response and not the researcher's assumptions.

Factor scores. By using the factors as a basis for analysis, it is possible to aggregate the scores for each statement contained in the factor and produce a factor score. An example of a factor produced from correlated statements is the Feeding Support Factor which arose from four statements in the postnatal care hospital questionnaire:

1. The midwives and nurses were helpful when I was feeding my baby.
2. I was helped to feel confident when I was feeding my baby.
3. The midwives and nurses seemed to understand what help I needed.
4. I needed more help in feeding my baby than I was given.

These four statements formed the factor. The mother's score might be:

Question 1 Agree   Score 4
Question 2 Disagree   Score 2
Question 3 Disagree   Score 2
Question 4 Agree   Score 2

In this case the factor score for this mother would be ten out of a possible maximum score of 20.

Factors that arose from the questionnaires.

1. Postnatal care in hospital (six factors):
   feeding support
   reaction to ward atmosphere
   physical well-being
   rest in hospital
   self-image related to feeding
   conflicting advice
2. Postnatal care in the community (four factors):
   support given by midwives
   continuity of advice
   rest/family support
   self-confidence
3. Emotional well-being, satisfaction with motherhood and family support questionnaire (seven factors)

The factor analysis identified five main factors related to the emotional well-being of the mothers. The factors identified were:

1. depression/mood disturbance
2. coping ability
3. anxiety

4. sleep/anxiety
5. self-confidence

It was decided to combine the scores on all five factors in order to produce an overall measure for the dependent variable, emotional well-being six weeks after delivery. The satisfaction with motherhood factor was formed from five of the original seven statements, and emerged as a highly correlated factor. The family support factor arose from the remaining five statements.

Further evaluation of maternal satisfaction with motherhood

A further measure was built into the six-week post-delivery assessment, and this was a rating scale based upon that designed by Broussard and Hartner (1971). This scale asked the mother to compare her baby's progress with that of the 'average' baby when the infant was six weeks old. The scores for the scale were used to rate the mother's perception of her baby as 'doing better than the average baby', 'about the same as the average baby', or 'worse than the average baby'.

Selection of sample, planning the study, gaining consent

The remaining task in designing the methods to be used for the research was to determine the target population, the size and selection of the sample, and the framework for data collection. The strategy was then subjected to a pilot study consisting of 30 mothers before the main study was undertaken.

It was also necessary to obtain the consent of the ethical committee in the areas selected for the study, and to gain the agreement of the midwives and obstetricians concerned. The consent of each mother involved was invited by an initial letter explaining the purpose of the study during the antenatal interview; it was then confirmed after delivery of the baby and before the post-delivery interview took place.

Target population. The target population was defined as women receiving maternity care from the National Health Service and booked for delivery in a consultant maternity hospital.

Sample. The sample was based on a cohort group from each of three maternity hospitals. Participants were selected from the antenatal records of women booked for delivery within a three month period who fulfilled the necessary sample criteria and who were willing to participate. During this preliminary selection process the following groups of women were excluded:

1. women with a history of infertility, previous stillbirth, or neonatal death, and any who had required admission to an antenatal ward

before the 36th week of pregnancy
2. women from Asian communities, and West Indian women who had not been born in this country. This was to reduce the effect of different cultural patterns and the problems of language difficulties.
3. women aged under 16 or over 40 at the time of booking, and any whose baby was to be adopted or the focus of a special care order.

Sample size. It was considered that a sample of 100 women from each hospital would provide sufficient numbers for a valid comparison of factors in the mother and factors in the postnatal care system that contributed to her emotional well-being and satisfaction with motherhood.

A total of 347 women were recruited from the antenatal records. Of the 320 mothers interviewed after delivery, 279 returned the six-week postnatal questionnaire, yielding a response rate of 87%. The data presented in this chapter relate to these 279 women.

A variety of non-parametric statistical methods were used to evaluate the relationship between the various events of childbirth and postnatal care, and the mother's emotional well-being and satisfaction with motherhood six weeks after the birth of the baby. These methods included the Spearman rank correlation, Mann–Whitney U test, and Kruskall–Wallis one-way analysis of variance.

These methods rank a series of observations or scores from the lowest to the highest in order to examine the correlation that may exist between two or more sets of scores, and to determine whether the rank order of scores given by mothers in two or more different groups is sufficiently different as to indicate that it is unlikely that they come from the same population, that is, that the difference between the two groups is statistically different (Siegel, 1956).

FINDINGS

Some details about the mothers in the sample

Marital status and social class. Of the mothers in the sample ($n = 279$), 88% were married or in a stable union; 10% were single, and 2% were separated or divorced. Thirty-one per cent were in Social Classes 1 and 2; 14% in Social Class 3 non-manual; 24% in Class 3 manual; and 26% were in Classes 4 and 5, with 4% unclassified.

Parity. Of the mothers in the sample, 35% were primigravidae; 42% were having their second baby; and the remaining 23% were having third or fourth babies.

Details of the labour and delivery. The onset of labour was spontaneous for 123 mothers (44%); induced for 97 mothers (35%); and 58 mothers (21%) had their labour accelerated by the use of oxytocinon.

The delivery was normal for 195 mothers (70%); 50 mothers (18%) had a forceps delivery; 29 (10%) were delivered by caesarean section and 4 women (1%) had a vaginal breech delivery.

The third stage of labour was normal for 257 mothers (92%). Nine babies (3.2%) needed to be transferred at birth to the special care baby unit but none of them required care in that unit for more than 48 hours.

Infant feeding. On the day of discharge from hospital, 162 mothers (58%) were breast feeding their baby; 93 mothers (33%) were bottle feeding; and the remaining 19 mothers from whom information was obtained were giving a combination of breast and bottle feeds (7%).

Defining degrees of emotional well-being and satisfaction with motherhood

Emotional well-being. Emotional well-being was measured by the score given by mothers to the 23 statements in the emotional well-being factor. The possible range of total scores was from 23 to 115; the scores recorded ranged from 48 to 108, with a mean score of 78.179, standard deviation 7.516. The scores were then grouped in order to define different levels of emotional well-being:

1. Emotional distress: 54 mothers (19.4%) who scored 68 or less were considered to be showing signs of emotional distress and depression.
2. Satisfactory emotional well-being: 196 mothers (70.3%) who scored between 69 and 91 were included in this group.
3. High emotional well-being: 30 mothers (10.8%) scored more than 92 and were considered to be very happy and satisfied.

These findings were consistent with those from previous studies of postnatal depression. The pattern of scoring of the mothers included in the low emotional well-being group showed a picture of depression, guilt and anxiety about the baby, which was reminiscent of that described by Pitt (1968).

Satisfaction with motherhood. The scores on this factor showed that the majority of women were satisfied and happy with motherhood six weeks after delivery. The factor was made up of five statements, making a possible total score of 5 to 25. The scores recorded were from 14 to 25, mean average 20.656, standard deviation 2.410. Only three mothers (1.1%) scored 14 or less and were considered to be dissatisfied with motherhood; 77 mothers (27.6%) scored between 15 and 19; and 199 mothers (71.3%) scored more than 20.

Factors which were related to maternal emotional well-being. Three main groups of factors were identified as having a highly significant relationship with emotional outcome. The details can be seen in Tables 8.1 and 8.2.

Table 8.1 Mothers' postnatal emotional well-being scores compared with their antenatal scores for trait anxiety (neuroticism) on the Eysenck Personality Inventory (Kruskall–Wallis one-way analysis of variance)

Emotional well-being scores	*Eysenck neuroticism scores*	
	no.	*mean rank score*
Low scores (emotional distress)	54	186.4
Satisfactory scores	187	125.7
High scores	27	91.6

Source: Compiled by the author.
N.B. Data were not available for 11 women

Anxiety and its effects. There was a highly significant relationship between trait anxiety measured on the Eysenck Personality Inventory at 36 weeks of pregnancy and the mother's emotional well-being six weeks after the birth ($p < 0.0001$). Trait anxiety also affected the mother's perception of events and self-confidence in the early postnatal weeks.

Stress related to life crises and postnatal care. The coping process was adversely affected by stress that arose from certain life crisis events and particular aspects of postnatal care.

Satisfaction with motherhood. There was a high correlation between the emotional well-being score and that for satisfaction with motherhood, which suggests that satisfaction with motherhood was not eroded by emotional distress, and that the mother's pleasure in her baby acted as a boost to emotional well-being and improved it. The satisfaction with motherhood score was found to have been affected by certain other factors related to the management of maternal care in hospital.

Maternal perception of the newborn. There was a high correlation between the mother's score for emotional well-being and satisfaction with motherhood, and her score on the Broussard-type scale, which recorded her perception of her baby's progress. Thirty-six women considered that their baby's progress at six weeks was worse than the 'average' baby. Broussard and Hartner's original work suggests that such a reaction at this early stage of parenting is an indicator of difficulties in the mother/child relationship.

Factors that were not related to emotional well-being included the following:

1. extroversion/introversion measured on the Eysenck Personality Inventory.

Table 8.2 Emotional well-being scores compared with life-events, self-image in feeding, rest in hospital, and satisfaction with motherhood and Broussard-type scores (Mann–Whitney and Kruskall–Wallis tests)

			Emotional well-being score	
		no.	mean rank score	
1.	*Life-Events*			
	a. Mothers reported marital tension	90	115.3	
	Mothers did not report marital tension	181	146.4	$p < 0.001$
	b. Mothers moved house	112	125.4	
	Mothers did not move house	160	144.3	$p < 0.05$
2.	*Self-Image in Feeding Scores*			
	Low scores	62	93.0	
	Satisfactory/high scores	206	147.0	$p < 0.001$
3.	*Rest in Hospital Scores*			
	Mothers reported too little sleep	118	125.7	
	Mothers did not report too little sleep	161	150.5	$p < 0.01$
4.	*Satisfaction with Motherhood*			
	Low scores	3	33.8	
	Moderate scores	77	124.7	
	High scores	199	147.5	$p < 0.01$
5.	*Broussard-type Scale*			
	Mothers considered baby's progress:			
	worse than the average baby	36	90.7	
	same as the average baby	127	140.7	
	better than the average baby	112	148.9	$p < 0.001$

Source: Compiled by the author.
Items 1–3 tested by Mann–Whitney U Test.
Items 4–5 tested by Kruskall–Wallis Tests.
N.B. Data in relation to items 1, 2 and 5 were not available for a few women (8 for life event a, 7 for life event b, 11 for self-image in feeding and 4 for views on baby's progress).

2. maternal separation from her own mother before the age of 11 years
3. the age and parity of the mother
4. the type of labour and delivery
5. the length of time the mother spent in hospital
6. the length of time for which the mother was visited by the community midwife

Testing the first hypothesis

Anxiety and its wide-ranging effects. The findings of the study upheld Lazarus' contention (1966, 1969) that anxiety has a powerful effect upon the coping process, emerging during the period of stress. Further analysis of the findings revealed an interactive relationship between trait anxiety and the mother's reactions in the postnatal period. Women who scored high trait anxiety at 36 weeks of pregnancy scored significantly lower scores for certain postnatal care factors, and these were:

1. reaction to ward atmosphere
2. physical well-being (in hospital)
3. self-confidence (at home)
4. perception of family support (at home)
5. perception of family support at six weeks postnatal

Anxious women found it less easy to relax and feel at home in the ward and their anxiety was shown in physical as well as emotional symptoms. There is no evidence to suggest that these reactions were due to the fact that these women received less care than the other mothers. A study of medical patients provides further evidence that people with high trait anxiety find it difficult to relax in hospital and may take some time to adjust (Wilson-Barnett, 1979).

The reports from the community midwives supported the mother's rating of her self-confidence when she returned home, and confirmed the effect of anxiety. Their reports, however, did not suggest that the women who scored low satisfaction with family support at this time did in fact receive less help than other mothers. It is likely that the mother's perception of family support, both when she first returned home with the baby and six weeks later, is in fact a symptom of her anxiety, expressing her lack of confidence in her own ability to cope with the baby.

It has been found that subjects with high trait anxiety react less well than those with low trait anxiety to learning situations in which their self-esteem is threatened (Glanzman and Laux, 1978). The findings of the study suggest that mothers who have high trait anxiety will require support for a longer period of time than other mothers before they become confident and competent in caring for their baby. This view is further confirmed by the study of Kumar and Robson (1978) who found that trait anxiety measured in the antenatal period was not a factor in the emotional status of women three months post-delivery. This suggests that the effects of trait anxiety upon the transition to motherhood is transitory and diminishes over time.

Life crisis stress. Pregnancy and childbirth are in themselves life/stress events requiring major adjustment. It would be foolish, however, to assume that these were the only life-events affecting the lives of parents. The mothers in the sample reported 456 life-events that had occurred during the year surrounding the birth of the baby.

Marital tension. It is perhaps not surprising to find that marital tension had a major effect upon emotional well-being. A relationship between marital conflict and depression has been demonstrated in many other studies of depression (Tod, 1964; Nuckolls *et al.*, 1972; Kumar and Robson, 1978; Oakley, 1980). It also emerged as a major cause of depression in women of any age in the study by Brown and Harris (1978). Mothers experiencing marital conflict or tension are deprived of a warm, confiding relationship and this can lead to feelings of vulnerability and lack of self-esteem or self-worth. Emotional support is therefore ineffective and the lack of such support may lead to apathy and depression.

Moving house. Although the statistical relationship between emotional well-being and the event of moving house was not as high as the other life-events (see Table 8.2), the number of women who had moved house in the year surrounding the pregnancy was surprisingly high (40% of the sample). This event was seen as a further contributory factor to emotional distress.

Antecedent factors uphold the first hypothesis. The antecedent factors of trait anxiety, marital stress, and moving house had a continuing effect upon the mother's adjustment to motherhood, and so the first hypothesis is upheld. This evidence, which is consistent with that from previous studies, highlights symptoms and situations that might be used by midwives to enable them to identify vulnerable women. Recently published work (Cox, 1986) has provided a useful scoring system that has been found to be highly valid in identifying women at risk of emotional disturbance during the postnatal period. The other factors that had a significant relationship with emotional well-being were not related to trait anxiety or to personal and family stress, but to the way in which care was provided by midwives during the postnatal period.

Testing the second hypothesis

Self-image in feeding. The mother's rating of her self-image in feeding in the early days in hospital expressed her feelings about her own competence in this important mothering skill. The self-image in feeding factor, which emerged from the postnatal care in hospital questionnaire, was quite separate from the feeding support factor, which assessed the mother's perception of the support given by midwives.

Self-criticism is a feature of depression (Beck *et al.*, 1961; Cox, 1986) and it might have been considered that women who were emotionally distressed at six weeks after delivery would look back upon their experience in hospital with jaundiced eyes, while those who felt happy and confident would have a more positive view of their self-image in feeding at that time. There was, however, considerable evidence that this was not the case, but rather that the self-image in feeding score reflected the mother's true feelings during the early postnatal period. Primiparae scored lower scores for self-image in feeding but they did not have significantly lower scores for emotional well-being. In fact, their emotional well-being was slightly higher than those of multiparae. The main evidence for the validity of the self-image in feeding score came from the hospital midwives' interview report. During that interview, the hospital midwives identified 54 mothers who were thought to have been 'unduly' distressed about feeding their baby and who had needed more help than the 'normal' mothers. The midwives considered that these women were distressed without any obvious cause. Six weeks later these women scored significantly lower scores for self-image in feeding. The picture emerges of two groups of women who showed anxiety about feeding their baby in the early postnatal period. For many of them, especially the primiparae, initial anxiety was replaced by growing confidence in skill and was not present six weeks later.

For certain others, however, the distress shown in the early days in the postnatal ward was a manifestation of emerging distress and of continuing problems of low self-esteem and conflict. This is further confirmed when we consider that the self-image in feeding score was significantly related to emotional well-being but not to satisfaction with motherhood.

Factors affecting self-image in feeding. Further analysis revealed a close relationship between the mother's scores on self-image in feeding, her report on the amount of rest she was able to gain in hospital, and the presence or absence of conflicting advice.

Conflicting advice. One hundred and nine women (39%) complained that they received conflicting advice from midwives and a number of these women also scored low self-image in feeding scores six weeks later. It could be expected that those who lack confidence and skill in feeding their baby will seek advice from those who care for them. The organization of care on the wards was based on a task – rather than client – allocation basis, and mothers were frequently cared for by a number of different midwives and other staff.

The nursing record frequently failed to record the details of advice that had been given and this made it difficult for a midwife to provide advice to a mother which built upon that previously given by a colleague. Conflicting advice has often been cited as a cause of dissatisfaction in maternity care (Clayton, 1979; Filshie *et al.*, 1981; Boyd and Sellers, 1982). Its effect is to reduce self-confidence further and may lead to women blaming themselves and assuming that they were at fault in being unable to deal adequately with their baby's feeding requirements. For certain vulnerable women, therefore, conflicting advice was yet another factor contributing to the spiral of lower self-esteem and consequent emotional distress ($p < 0.01$).

Lack of sleep in hospital. Another stress factor that contributed to low self-image ($p < 0.01$) and had a direct correlation with emotional well-being ($p < 0.01$) was lack of sleep in hospital. One hundred and fourteen mothers (41%) recorded low satisfaction with their rest in hospital and it was found that the primary cause was the lack of sleep at night. Further analysis revealed that this was more marked in the two hospitals that operated a 24-hour 'rooming-in' of mothers and babies.

A number of studies have shown that subjects deprived of the deeper stages of sleep rapidly become depressed and lethargic and lose their efficiency in carrying out manual skills (Weinmann, 1981). Lack of sleep is a frequent complaint of hospital patients; it is not easy to sleep in a strange environment that is disturbed by unusual noise and lights. Disturbance is even more likely in a ward with newborn babies crying throughout the night. Bernal (1972) reported a peak of crying of babies between midnight and 6.00 a.m. Other surveys of satisfaction with maternity care reveal a high degree of complaint about the lack of sleep caused by 'rooming-in' policies (Clayton, 1979; Filshie *et al.*, 1981; Boyd and Sellers, 1982). A comparative study by Cox (1974) found that 40% of mothers whose baby stayed with them through the night complained of too little sleep, and Draramraj *et al.* (1981) found that there were many factors that influenced mother's choice of whether to 'room-in' or not. Both Cox and Draramraj concluded that the maternal choice should be the deciding factor. Klaus and Kennel (1976, 1982) recommend that babies should be kept by their mother for long periods throughout the day and brought to them for feeding at night. It is unfortunate that in spite of all this evidence, many maternity hospitals continue to practise 24-hour rooming-in in a routine and indiscriminate manner.

Maternal perception of the newborn. The original study by Broussard and Hartner (1971) indicated that mothers with poor self-image regarded their baby as 'difficult' more often than other mothers. Other studies have shown a relationship between low self-esteem in the mother and continuing problems in mother/child relationships leading to child abuse (Lynch *et al.*, 1976; Rosen and Stein, 1980). The study by Lynch *et al.* is particularly interesting because, as in the study being reported, it was found that midwives in the maternity hospitals had identified the early problems of mothering, which were later found to be significant when the children of those mothers were considered to be at risk of non-accidental injury. The results of the study indicate that conflicting advice and lack of sleep in hospital were highly stressful factors that reduced self-confidence and self-image in feeding and contributed to emotional distress. The further relationship between that distress and the mother's perception of her newborn baby is particularly disturbing. It must be acknowledged, however, that the mother's self-esteem was not measured prior to delivery and the self-image in feeding factor may therefore reflect a number of women whose self-esteem was already low. The large numbers of women, however, who complained about rest in hospital (41% of the sample) and conflicting advice (39%) of the sample) serve to underline the effect that such stress had upon a large number of women. It also upholds the second hypothesis that the way care is given by midwives will have an effect upon women's emotional reactions to the changes that follow the birth of a child.

Satisfaction with motherhood. Satisfaction with motherhood was the secondary dependent variable and, as has already been explained, had a positive effect upon emotional well-being, boosting morale and enriching the adjustment process. Further analysis revealed that many of the factors that affected emotional well-being did not have a similar effect upon satisfaction with motherhood.

Factors that were not related to satisfaction with motherhood. Trait anxiety did not affect satisfaction with mother-hood. The age and parity of the mother, and choice of feeding method did not affect satisfaction with motherhood. Mothers who had a low score for self-image in feeding, and those who were seen to be distressed about feeding their baby while in hospital, did not score any less satisfaction with motherhood than other mothers. Although lack of rest as related to the patterns of 'rooming-in' of babies and mothers affected emotional well-being, it did not have a similar effect on satisfaction with mother-hood, and there was no significant difference in the levels of satisfaction with motherhood of the mothers in the three different hospitals. This indicates that the practice of putting babies into the nursery at night at one of the three hospitals did not have a detrimental effect upon the developing mother/child relationship. These results lead one to conclude that satisfaction with motherhood is a distinct and stable matrix of feel-ings and motivation that arise from a different source from those affecting the coping process.

Factors that did have a relationship with satisfaction with motherhood.

Mother's reported feelings after delivery. During the post-delivery interview, women were asked to record their feelings imme-diately after delivery. A small number of women who expressed themselves as 'disappointed', or 'too tired to care' scored significantly lower levels of satisfaction with motherhood six weeks after delivery. Those who described themselves as 'gloriously happy' at delivery showed very much higher satisfaction with motherhood six weeks later than any of the others. There was no evidence that the mother's feelings imme-diately after the delivery were affected by the type of labour or delivery she had experienced.

Feeding the baby in the first hour after delivery. There was, however, evidence that the giving and receiving of a feed in the first hour after delivery enhanced the mother's pleasure in her achievement and had an effect upon her continuing satisfaction with motherhood. Mothers who fed their baby within the first hour of delivery recorded more positive feelings at this time and the highest level of satisfaction with motherhood six weeks later (see Table 8.3).

A number of studies have focused upon the contact between the mother and the baby during the first hour after delivery and have demonstrated the beneficial effects that a period of mutual physical and eye contact has upon the developing mother/child relationship (Klaus and Kennell, 1970; Klaus *et al.*, 1972; Kennell *et al.*, 1975; Leiderman and Seashore, 1975). The giving of a feed allows a mother a period of uninterrupted time during the first hour after birth, and by facilitating the *en face* position, allows the eye contact that is known to have a beneficial effect.

It might be supposed that mothers who had had a difficult delivery would be less likely to feed their baby, but this was not so. Forty per cent of women who had a forceps delivery fed their baby during the first hour compared with 45% of those who had a normal delivery. The major reason underlying whether or not a mother fed her baby depended upon her choice of breast and bottle feeding and upon the management of care in the delivery suite (see Table 8.4).

It can be seen that younger mothers and those in Social Classes 3 manual, 4 and 5 fed their baby in the delivery suite less frequently than those in the other groups. This difference was not entirely due to a more frequent choice of bottle feeding among these women. The reason may lie in the fact that these women are less likely to be articulate and

Table 8.3 Mothers' birth feelings and satisfaction with motherhood scores classified by time of first feed to baby (Mann–Whitney U Test; corrected for ties)

Time that mother fed baby	Birth feelings (24 hours after birth)	
	no.	mean rank score
Within first hour of birth	112	151.3
More than one hour after birth	164	129.8
	$z = 2.2769$; $p < 0.02$	

	Satisfaction with motherhood (six weeks after birth)	
	no.	mean rank score
Within one hour of birth	113	151.6
More than one hour after birth	165	131.2
	$z = 2.0921$; $p < 0.03$	

Source: Compiled by the author.
N.B. Data on birth feelings were not available for 3 women, and on satisfaction with motherhood for one woman.

Table 8.4 Choice of feeding method, age and social class of mothers, by whether baby was fed within one hour of birth (Chi-square tests)

	Fed baby within one hour of birth		Did not feed baby within one hour of birth		Total	
	no.	%	*no.*	%	*no.*	%
Total sample	109	40.1	163	59.9	272	100
Feeding Method						
Breast	93	58.1	67	41.9	160	100
Bottle	16	14.3	96	85.7	112	100
$p < 0.0001$ (1 d.f.)						
Age						
17–20 years	4	12.9	27	87.1	31	100
21–29 years	70	42.9	93	57.1	163	100
30–39 years	38	45.2	46	54.8	84	100
$p < 0.01$ (2 d.f.)						
Social Class						
Classes 1 and 2	44	51.8	41	48.2	85	100
Class 3 non-manual	20	51.3	19	48.7	39	100
Class 3 manual	25	36.8	43	63.2	68	100
Classes 4 and 5	19	26.8	52	73.2	71	100
Unclassified	4	36.4	7	63.6	11	100
$p < 0.01$ (4 d.f.)						

Source: Compiled by the author.
N.B. Data were not available for a few women in relation to each of the variables in the table (7 for whether baby fed within one hour after birth, 7 for feeding method, 1 for age and 5 for social class).

demanding in their desire to feed their baby as soon as possible after delivery. This view is substantiated by the fact that although all three hospitals included in the study had policies that mothers should be encouraged to put the baby to the breast as soon after birth as possible, in fact 41.9% of breastfeeding mothers were not given an opportunity to feed their baby in the delivery suite. This suggests that in the busy atmosphere of the labour suite, midwives may overlook the need to provide a time for mothers and babies to delight in each other.

Attention must also be drawn to the needs of bottle feeding women, and it is a matter of regret that many delivery suites do not yet provide an opportunity for such women to spend time feeding their baby.

There is a need to recognize this important period in the first hour after delivery as a fourth stage of labour, which should be managed as carefully as the first three. Midwives have a particular role to play in changing the management of delivery suites in order to enhance mother/child relationships.

CONCLUSIONS

The findings of the study illustrated the complex and dynamic situation surrounding adjustment to motherhood, and the many factors that inter-act with each other to have an effect upon it. Although the outcome of adjustment to motherhood measured at six weeks postnatal was strongly influenced by personality and family stress, there was considerable evidence that the management of care in the delivery suite and in the post-natal wards also had an important effect upon the adjustment process. These factors may be seen as those that Caplan described as 'loading the dice' in favour of a good or bad emotional outcome.

The fact that midwives were able to identify mothers who were experiencing distress indicates that this early recognition of vulnerable women could be used to identify those in need of increased and extended support. Conflicting advice and lack of rest in hospital had a negative effect upon emotional outcome and these problems could be overcome by changes in the management of care.

Postnatal care provided by midwives in the Health Service is one part of the whole interactive framework of support which a woman requires if she is to make a successful and happy adjustment to motherhood. The mother's personality and her previous experiences are largely fixed and impervious to change. The situation of marital tension and lack of family support may also not be amenable to change by midwives.

The factor that is amenable to change, however, is the service given by midwives, health visitors, doctors and all those concerned with the care of mothers and babies. Midwives in particular have much to contribute to the emotional health of mothers and babies. This contribution could be made by improving the flexibility of approach to the care of women in the postnatal period, identifying those most at risk (Cox, 1986), and spend-ing time during the postnatal period in enabling women to adjust and adapt in a way that is right for them, helping them to develop their mothering skills at a pace that is consistent with their needs. Affonso (1984) discusses ways in which those caring for women in the postnatal period can enable them to internalize their feelings and lead to increased understanding.

The overriding principle in helping mothers to gain confidence in themselves and their ability to care for their baby lies in providing encouragement and praise. If all goes well, the mother becomes more confident, but nothing interferes more with the growth of empathy between a mother and her baby than failure and criticism (McKeith, 1966). The close contact that exists between mothers and midwives, especially during labour and the early postnatal period, gives midwives a unique opportunity to observe and to influence a mother's response to the demands that motherhood makes upon her.

There is a need to review critically the patterns of postnatal care that currently exist and provide a more flexible approach to this important, but generally neglected, aspect of maternity care. By reducing the incidence of postnatal depression and distress – which is currently cited as affecting between 10 and 20% of all mothers – midwives, health visitors, obstetricians and general practitioners have an opportunity to improve the mental health of the nation and enhance and enrich mother/child relationships to a considerable degree.

REFERENCES

Affonso, D.D. (1984) Postpartum depression. In Field, P.A. (ed.), *Perinatal nursing*, Churchill Livingstone, Edinburgh.

Ball, J.A. (1983) The effect of the present patterns of maternity care upon the emotional needs of mothers, with particular reference to the postnatal period. Unpublished thesis, Faculty of Medicine, Manchester University.

Ball, J.A. (1987) *Reactions to motherhood: The role of postnatal care.* Cambridge University Press, Cambridge.

Beck, A.T., Ward. C.H., Mendelson, M., Mock, J. and Erbaugh, J. (1961) An inventory for measuring depression. *Archives of General Psychiatry, 4,* 561–71.

Bernal, J. (1972) Crying during the first ten days of life and maternal response. *Developmental Medicine and Child Neurology, 4,* 362–72.

Boyd, C. and Sellers, L. (1982) *The British way of birth.* Pan Books, London.

Broussard, E.R. and Hartner, M.S.S. (1971) Further considerations regarding maternal perception of the newborn. In Jerome, J. (ed.), *Exceptional infant: Studies in abnormality,* Brunner-Mazel, New York, pp. 432–49.

Brown, G. and Harris, T. (1978) *Social origins of depression: A study of psychiatric disorder in women.* Tavistock, London.

Brown, W.A. (1979) *Psychological care during pregnancy and the post-natal period.* Raven Press, New York.

Caplan, G. (1964) *Principles of preventative psychiatry.* Tavistock, London.

Caplan, G. (1969) An approach to community mental health. Tavistock, London.

Clayton, S. (1979) *Maternity care: Some patients' views.* Survey carried out by Newcastle Community Health Council in Newcastle-upon-Tyne Hospitals.

Cox, B.S. (1974) Rooming in. *Nursing Times* (August), 1246.

Cox, J.L., Connor, Y. and Kendell, R.E. (1982) Prospective study of the psychiatric disorders of childbirth. *British Journal of Psychiatry, 140,* 111–17.

Cox, J.L. (1986) *Postnatal Depression, A Guide for Health Professionals,* Churchill Livingstone, Edinburgh.

Draramraj, C., Siac, G., Kierney, C.M., Harper, R.C., Pareck, A. and Weissman, B. (1981) Observations on maternal preference for rooming-in Harper Facilities. *Paediatrics, 67* (5), 638–40.

Erikson, E.H. (1963) *Childhood and society* (2nd edn). Norton, New York.

Eysenk, H.J. and Eysenck, S.B.G. (1968) *Manual of the Eysenck Personality Questionnaire.* Hodder and Stoughton, Kent.

Filshie, S., Williams, J., Osbourn, M., Senior, O.E., Symonds, E.M. and Backett, E.M. (1981) Postnatal care in hospitals – Time for a change. *International Journal of Nursing Studies, 18* (2), 89–95.

Frommer, E.A. and O'Shea, G. (1973) Antenatal identification of women liable to have problems in managing their infants. *British Journal of Psychiatry*, *123*, 149–56.

Glanzman, P. and Laux, L. (1978) The effects of trait anxiety and two kinds of stressors on state anxiety and performance. In Spielburger, C. and Sarason, I.G. (eds), *Stress and anxiety*, vol. 3, John Wiley & Sons, New York.

Holmes, T.H. and Rahe, R.H. (1967) Social readjustment rating scale. *Journal of Psychosomatic Research*, *11*, 219.

Kennell, J.H., Trause, M.A. and Klaus, M.H. (1975) Evidence for a sensitive period in the human mother. In Porter, E and O'Connor, M. (eds), *Parent–Infant interaction*, Ciba Foundation Symposium no. 33, Associated Scientific Publishers, Amsterdam, pp. 87–101.

Klaus, M.H. and Kennell, J.H. (1970) Human maternal behaviour at first contact with her young. *Pediatrics*, *46* (2), 187–92.

Klaus, M.H., Jerauld, R., Kreger, N.C., McAlpine, W., Steffa, M. and Kennell, J.H. (1972) Maternal attachment: Importance of the first post-partum days. *New England Journal of Medicine*, *286*, 460–3.

Klaus, M.H. and Kennell, J.H. (1976) *Maternal–Infant bonding*. C.V. Mosby, St. Louis.

Klaus, M.H. and Kennell, J.H. (1982) *Parent–Infant bonding*. C.V. Mosby, St. Louis.

Klaus, M.H., Trause, M.A. and Kennell, J.H. (1978) Does human maternal behaviour after delivery show a characteristic pattern? In Porter, E. and O'Connor, M. (eds), *Parent–Infant interaction*, Ciba Foundation Symposium no. 33, Associated Scientific Publishers, Amsterdam, pp. 69–85.

Kumar, R. and Robson, K. (1978) Neurotic disturbance during pregnancy and the puerperium. In Sandler, M. (ed.) *Mental illness in pregnancy and the puerperium*, Oxford University Press, Oxford, pp. 40–51.

Kumar, R. and Robson, K. (1984) A prospective study of emotional disorders in childbearing women. *British Journal of Psychiatry*, *144*, 33–47.

Lazarus, R.S. (1966) *Psychological stress and the coping process*. McGraw-Hill, New York.

Lazarus, R.S. (1969) *Patterns of adjustment and human effectiveness*. McGraw-Hill, New York.

Leiderman, P.H. and Seashore, M.J. (1975) Mother-infant separation: Some delayed consequences. In Porter, E. and O'Connor, M. (eds), *Parent–Infant interaction*, Ciba Foundation Symposium no. 33, Associated Scientific Publishers, Amsterdam, pp. 213–39.

Likert, R. (1932) A technique for the measurement of attitudes. *Archives of Psychology*, *140*.

Lynch, M.A., Roberts, J. and Gordon, M. (1976) Child abuse: Early warning in the maternity hospital. *Developmental Medicine and Child Neurology*, *18*, 759–66.

McKeith, R. (1966) How can we help the mother to adapt to her child? *Proceedings of the Royal Society of Medicine*, *59*, 1013–18.

Nuckolls, C.B., Cassell, J. and Kaplan, B.H. (1972) Psycho-social assets, life-crises and the prognosis of pregnancy. *American Journal of Epidemiology*, *95*, 431–34.

Oakley, A. (1980) *Women confined*. Martin Robertson, Oxford.

Oppenheim, A.N. (1966) *Questionnaire design and attitude measurement*. Heinemann, London.

Pitt, B. (1968) 'Atypical' depression following childbirth. *British Journal of*

Psychiatry, 114, 1325–35.

Rapoport, R., Rapoport, R.N. and Strelitz, Z. (1977) *Fathers, mothers and others.* Routledge & Kegan Paul, London.

Rosen, B. and Stein, M.T. (1980) Children and abusive women. *American Journal of Diseases of Childhood, 134.*

Siegel, S. (1956) *Non-parametric statistics for the behavioural sciences.* McGraw Hill, London.

Stopher, P.R. and Meyburg, A.H. (1979) *Survey sampling and multivariate analysis for social scientists and engineers.* Lexington Books, Lexington, Mass.

Stott, D.H. (1973) Follow-up study from birth of the effect on prenatal stresses. *Developmental Medicine and Child Neurology, 15,* 770–87.

Tod, E.D.M. (1964) Puerperal depression: A prospective epidemiology study. *Lancet, II,* 1264.

Treece, K.W. and Treece, J.W. (1977) *Elements of research in nursing.* C.V. Mosby, St. Louis.

Weinmann, J. (1981) *An outline of psychology as applied to medicine.* John Wright & Sons Ltd., Bristol.

Wilson-Barnett, J. (1979) *Stress in hospital: Patients' psychological reactions to illness and health care.* Churchill Livingstone, Edinburgh.

CHAPTER NINE

Midwives' and mothers' perceptions of motherhood

Maureen Laryea

The postnatal period, especially for the first-time mother, is an important period of transition, marking the end of pregnancy and the start of motherhood. Assumption of this new status may be characterized by manifold difficulties: the woman has to fulfil the obligations of her new status, learn how to relate to the baby who is unable to communicate verbally, as well as coping with the physical and emotional changes occurring in her own body. It is an event influenced by biological and physiological variables as well as social and cultural norms. As Strauss (1962) pointed out, the passage from one status to another is often highly institutionalized, particularly when the transition is typical for most members of a group. Thus in some societies, most women are expected to leave school, take a job, get married and become a mother. These status passages are governed by relatively clear rules that indicate when the change should be made and by whom. There are prescribed sequences of steps that the person must go through to complete the passage and there are regularized actions that must be carried out by various relevant others in order that this passage is actually accomplished.

With regard to the transition to motherhood in pre-industrial society, the relevant others would include family, friends and neighbours, as well as local women who act as midwives. Oakley (1977) commented that pre-industrial societies generally show a degree of cohesion and a sense of community not often found in modern industrial society, and there is usually consensus in both the ideology and the practice of childbirth. It is possible that this congruity minimizes tension between the recipient of care and her care-givers.

In western society, however, the relevant others for the childbearing woman include professional care-givers (primarily doctors and midwives) as well as family and friends. A number of studies have shown that the beliefs held by the former about the nature and management of childbirth and the meaning of motherhood may be incongruent with those held by the women for whom they care (Comaroff, 1977; Hart, 1977; Graham and Oakley, 1981; Romalis, 1985). This in turn may generate tension and conflict, particularly for the recipient of care.

The disorganization of the woman/couple's lifestyle following child-birth has been viewed by some as a crisis (Le Masters, 1957; Hobbs, 1965; Dyers, 1965). Other studies, however (Rapoport, 1963; Rossi, 1974), while not underplaying the crisis occurring around this period of childbirth, consider it to be a normal event, albeit one requiring readjust-ment. Raphael (1975) states that it is the people who are in contact with the new mother in the early phase of this transition period, who are influ-ential in helping her accept her new status and cope with and adjust to its demands. As one of the first groups of professionals to come into contact with the new mother, midwives have a crucial role in this process. This chapter is concerned with similarities and differences in midwives' and women's views of motherhood, the needs of newly delivered women, and the midwives' methods of assessing these needs. The data were collected in the course of a project that sought to examine the care given by midwives to primiparous women and their baby in the first month postnatally (Laryea, 1980).

METHODS

The data were collected by means of observation and interview over a period of 12 months in one ward in each of two hospitals. The rationale for using these methods was to allow the researcher to investigate whether there was a difference between what was reported and what actually happened in the ward. Another aim was to consider what effect the differences in the midwives' and mothers' perceptions of motherhood would have on the care given to and received by postpartum women.

The sample

The sample was composed of 44 primiparous women who had delivered a live baby. The age of the subjects studied ranged between 16 and 36 years. Exclusion criteria were as follows:

1. All unmarried women were considered unsuitable as they may not have been involved in the care of their baby pending adoption.
2. Women were excluded if their baby had major congenital abnormal-ities, they delivered a pre-term baby or if their baby died in the course of the study.

All the women who satisfied the above criteria were approached follow-ing their admission to the eight-bed ward used for the study and invited to take part.

The midwives providing the care were also studied. 20 hospital midwives giving postnatal care during both day and night and 20 community midwives giving after-care to the women in this study. The age range of the midwives was 25 to 49 years. The investigator pledged to keep anonymous and confidential the names of participants, hospitals and health authority used in the study.

Observation

Categories of observation research. Gold (1958) identified four categories of observation technique, ranging from complete participant to complete observer. However, other researchers (e.g. Stacey, 1969) subscribe to the view that there are only two main categories – complete participant and complete observer – the others being subtypes. The fieldworker may find his or her position and activities shifting through time from one to another of these positions within the same observation session (Junker, 1960).

The complete participant observer's true identity and purpose are unknown to those whom she observes, for she interacts with them and participates fully in whatever areas of their lives are accessible to her so that she may learn about the people she is observing. The complete observer, on the other hand, has no social interaction with the observed. Between these two categories are the participant-as-observer, where the role of the observer is known by the observed and interaction between them occurs, and the observer-as-participant, which is used in the situation of formal observation.

The disadvantage of the complete participant role is that the investigator may 'go native' and find it almost impossible to report the findings of her study. The investigator considered this a risk because of her professional background as a midwife. While the complete participant role offers possibilities of learning about aspects of behaviour that might otherwise be overlooked by a field observer, it places the investigator in what Denzin (1970) has called a 'pretended role', calling for a delicate balance between the demands of this pretended role and self. Furthermore, the investigator faces the ethical problem of observing and recording data without the participant's knowledge and permission.

The complete observer risks misinterpreting the situation observed since she does not fully engage in it and, because she does not interact with informants, the chances are that she will be seen by them as being aloof. As this study involved continuous observations over time, the category of observer as participant was inappropriate; her contact with the informant is brief and so she is more likely to misunderstand the informant and to be misunderstood by the informant (Denzin, 1970).

The category adopted in the study was that of participant-as-observer, since this meant that the investigator was free to form relationships with the subjects, so that they served both as respondents and as informants. A participant-as-observer is involved in ongoing social processes in the research setting and the negotiation of a role that is acceptable to the subjects being observed.

The observation fieldwork. As this observer had to gain acceptance by both mothers and midwives and be able to move freely among them, a marginal role was adopted. Some unpleasant feelings derived from playing this role were experienced, for example, when the observer was in the company of women who expressed strong views about certain members of staff and was then seen by those same mothers to be having tea with the staff members they had criticized.

Initially members of staff became anxious when the observer took notes at the scene of action. Gradually, however, they accepted this as part of the observer's work, thus confirming Fox's (1976) suggestion that the situation goes back to normal when the observer is established. Observations were carried out for four to five hours a day and a complete narrative of what happened was produced. For example, when the observer watched staff helping a woman to breastfeed her baby, a full description of the activity was recorded. Incidents that were expressions of attitudes, actions by individuals or groups, and conversations were recorded fully. Occasionally it was considered that note-taking at the scene of action would interfere with the action, for example, when the observer accompanied the family planning nurse during her ward rounds as the discussions that took place were considered too 'sensitive'.

Initially, it was difficult to remain in the role of observer while midwives and staff were working under pressure. In order to overcome this, the observer engaged in some menial task that did not involve maternal care, for example, finding people to answer the telephone, passing on messages or finding a midwife when a woman needed one. The observer attended meals with staff and had the opportunity to use the staff rest room at lunchtime. The relationship that the observer had established with staff meant that she was the recipient of confidences about other members of staff and about various conflicts between midwives and doctors that were frequently discussed in the staff rest room. Although the women's stay in hospital was of short duration, being with them for long periods each day resulted in the observer getting to know more about them than did the staff. However, because the observer did not want the women to respond to her as a midwife and seek information pertaining to midwifery care, she dissociated herself from the midwife's role by not wearing a uniform or engaging in midwifery duties, and by sitting and talking with the women in the dayroom.

The women regularly asked for information pertaining to baby feeding but it was not possible to respond and in such instances, women were directed to the staff for information. Difficulty also arose when both women and midwives sought the observer's views in discussions that occurred in the ward. For example, when one midwife told a woman to put her baby back into its cot because she would spoil it, the mother said 'Can you tell me, nurse, at what stage does a baby get spoiled?' The midwife replied, 'I'm telling you, you'll spoil her before you know it; she will soon know that if she cries, you'll pick her up!' Woman: 'That does not answer my question.' At this point, the midwife and the other woman in the ward said to the observer, 'What do you think?' The views of the observer were congruent with those of the woman but to have expressed them would have been seen as taking sides, leading to possible reprisals. Therefore, the observer said that she could not express her views on the incident and this was accepted by both parties.

On occasion, when the urge to revert to the role of midwife was intense, the observer either left the room for a while or took action. For example, one woman was worried because her baby (two days old) was vomiting and had jittery movements. She asked a nursing auxiliary to look at the baby. the woman was assured that occasionally all babies have jittery movements and that it was because her baby was dreaming. But the woman did not appear convinced. Later the observer looked at the baby and called a midwife to deal with the situation. This incident was handled in such a way that neither the nursing auxiliary nor the woman was aware that the observer had reported the incident, and thus possible unpleasantness in the ward was avoided.

This incident highlights the main ethical problem that confronts the investigator involved in the participant-as-observer role – that of making decisions about whether and how to intervene in a clinical situation without such action being interpreted as 'interference' by the subjects involved. There was an advantage in the observer also being a midwife, in that those being observed (midwives) saw her as being conversant with the midwifery care of women and were therefore less inhibited in their actions and comments. Also, because the observer was no longer working within the National Health Service, it was easy to ask questions without being viewed with suspicion.

At the beginning of the study, the observer did not fully appreciate the impact of observing, from a different perspective, those activities in which she had once participated and which now appeared to be at variance with her own values and beliefs. The observer constantly reminded herself that the purpose of the study was to describe and explain events, not to pass judgement.

Interviews. While the observation technique yielded data pertinent to the study in that it showed how the process of midwifery was effected, the method nevertheless was inadequate in obtaining information on the midwives' and women's perceptions of motherhood. Therefore, formal interviews and informal discussions were used to collect these data. Since contact and the building of relationships with both midwives and the women were already established during the observation periods, it was to the researcher's advantage to maintain this personal contact rather than sever it by using questionnaires, which are considered to be impersonal (Selltiz *et al.*, 1966). The interviews offered the benefit of recording not only what the respondent said but also how it was said, thus highlighting areas of concern, satisfaction, dissatisfaction and anger.

The interview schedules contained closed and open questions to encourage the interviewees to express themselves fully. This form of questioning allows the interviewee to develop her own views. Probing and prompting techniques were also used to ensure that questions were answered in depth. However, caution was used so as not to introduce bias by the overuse of these techniques.

Sequence of interviews. The women were interviewed on three occasions in the following order:

1. The first interview took place in hospital, the day prior to being transferred to the care of the community midwife. The main aim of this interview was to obtain information on the woman's views of midwifery care received in hospital, her perceived needs as well as her views of motherhood.
2. The second interview was held between the tenth and the twelfth day following the birth of the baby. The aim of this interview was to find out how the mother coped at home, how she saw her needs, her personal concerns and the difficulties since returning home, as well as her view of motherhood.
3. The final interview was held when the baby was between 28 and 30 days old. This allowed the woman to give a more comprehensive view of motherhood in the first month after childbirth.

The midwives in hospital and in the community were interviewed following the completion of the mother's interviews and observations.

DATA ANALYSIS

Data were obtained from observations, formal interviews, informal discussions, information from the women's and babies' medical records, midwifery reports and letters of referral. The data collected from observation and from informal discussions were indexed and labelled, each entry having a code number referring to major topics. The major topics included the midwives' views of the needs of women, the mothers' views of their needs and the teaching of baby care skills. Each of these major categories was broken down into subcategories, for example, 'the needs of newly delivered mothers' included the subcategories 'mothers' and 'midwives' views on motherhood; 'physical care'; and 'emotional care'. These subcategories were further divided into topics. The data were filed in chronological order, thus making possible a relatively quick check of data on a given point.

Data analysis was undertaken concurrently from the time the first data were collected. By constantly re-analysing data previously collected, various categories as well as views held by both the women and the midwives emerged and recurred. For example, there were women who breastfed and those who bottle fed their baby. The identification of these categories led the observer to collect data on how these two groups were given help by midwives, together with the midwives' views on the kind of help needed by each group. An example of the views held by midwives of the woman's ability to cope with her baby and adjust to motherhood was evident in the labelling used by midwives; terms such as 'copers', 'late copers' or 'problem mothers' were applied. The observer had to seek information substantiating the existence of such qualities and characteristics in these groups.

Constant re-analysis of data necessitated the formulation of new propositions; while at the same time, looking for negative cases which would warrant the re-formulation of existing propositions, or the rejection of others. For example, a proposition was made that all women would receive adequate supervision during the baby's feeding times until they were discharged from hospital. While data were being collected on how women were supervised, it became apparent that greater specificity was required, stating the number of people involved in supervising the woman at each feed, the information imparted to the woman during supervision, as well as the categorization of women according to the method of feeding they had chosen, since this affected the length of time the woman was supervised.

In this way, propositions were refined as categories of women evolved from data associated with supervision during baby feeding times. New data were sought as a result of refined propositions, which involved re-analysis of the mass of data collected earlier in the study, engaging in what Glaser and Strauss (1967) called 'collecting data from collected data'.

A quantitative analysis was performed on the structured questions from the interview schedules and on the information from the demonstrations of infant-orientated skills. The open-ended responses from interview schedules were typed out so that they could be sorted into appropriate categories. These were then rewritten, resorted and redefined until sets of categories emerged with as few unclassified answers as possible. The data obtained from the two hospitals differed little and are therefore presented together in the next section unless otherwise stated.

FINDINGS AND IMPLICATIONS

The data from this small-scale study suggested that there was a fundamental difference in the perspectives used by the midwives and mothers who took part in this study in defining the meaning of motherhood. In defining motherhood, the midwives used and emphasized the biological and medical aspects of motherhood, seeing it as a normal process in a woman's life cycle and an indication that she has achieved physical maturity. The midwives acknowledged that this particular stage in a woman's life cycle brought with it the added responsibility of looking after a new infant. Therefore it was important that, following delivery, the new mother should be in a good physical state to enable her to undertake her new responsibilities. The view that care given to women in the postnatal period largely focuses on physical aspects (Reeder *et al.*, 1971) is confirmed by this study.

The mothers, however, viewed motherhood from a different perspective; for them, its meaning extended beyond the biological act of reproduction and the birth process. For although they equated motherhood with the achievement of femininity and were relieved by the knowledge that they were able to bear a child, the main emphasis was placed on their acquisition of a new social role. The social perspective of motherhood was missing in the midwives' perspectives, yet it was this social aspect that the women stressed.

According to these women, their new role gave them a senior status, a sense of belonging and feelings of recognition. One statement included the following:

> Everybody behaves differently towards you from the time they know you're expecting a baby; your neighbours show concern, your husband, family and friends; you just feel you are held in high regard.

The acquisition of a new social status was a boost to their self-image and confidence; they expected that midwives would recognize their achievement and respond in a way similar to that shown by friends and family. When the expected responses were not elicited from midwives, the women were disappointed and thus tension prevailed.

The situation is compounded when a women is delivered in hospital because she acquires two roles simultaneously, that is, the motherhood role and the 'patient' role. These two roles are antagonistic. The former is a 'progressive' stage in the woman's life cycle, and is considered to be fundamental to the woman's self-concept (Hart, 1977). Patienthood, however, can be viewed as a regressive status, its incumbent losing her locus of control. The biological and medical perspectives of motherhood allow the midwife to place the woman in the patienthood role while the woman herself uses the social definition of motherhood.

Conflicts arising from the use of different perspectives

If two individuals hold different views about a particular situation or role, their expectations may also differ and this may lead to frustration and tension (Freidson, 1975). Because the midwives and the women used different perspectives to view motherhood, frustration and tension were evident, particularly on the part of the women. These feelings arose because the women's expectations were not realized and their needs were not fully met by the midwives.

Some of the major areas that generated a great deal of tension in the women were in taking responsibility for the baby, in building a relationship with the baby, and the new mother's own needs.

Taking up responsibility. Although midwives made the statement that motherhood brought with it the added responsibility for women of looking after their new baby, the midwives nevertheless took full responsibility for both woman and baby throughout their stay in hospital. Women were told when to change their baby, when to feed, and when to put him or her down. Thus, while the woman and her baby remain in hospital, all decisions pertaining to the welfare of the baby are made by the midwife; yet on discharge home, the woman must assume full responsibility immediately. One midwife said:

> You see, in hospital we take the responsibility [meaning taking decisions about infant well-being] but we do allow the mother to carry out all the tasks concerned with the care.

This statement indicates that women in hospital do not fulfil all obligations of their new role. As a result of this, some women were disappointed. Thus the woman must concern herself with carrying out the practical activities of baby care, without also being an active participant in the decision-making concerning her baby's welfare.

The midwives' approach was incongruent with the women's views of motherhood as a senior status; the women perceived that their care-givers did not appreciate or recognize their new status and they felt that in hospital they were being 'treated like children'.

It could be argued that not all women would wish to make decisions on their baby's behalf. However, a joint approach towards decision-making would be a better proposition since the woman is the principal decision-maker when she returns home. The data showed that one of the main difficulties faced by women on returning home concerned making decisions about baby care and assuming responsibility for decisions made. While it is acknowledged that there is a need to initiate the woman into her new role, the initiation should be carried out in a way that will boost her self-image and ego; otherwise there is the danger of 'bruising' both, and the woman may take a long time to recover from it.

Building up the mother–baby relationship. Caplain (1961) pointed out that a number of women develop a relationship with their fetus *in utero* and this relationship is developed further after birth. In some women, childbirth itself marks the beginning of the mother-baby relationship and how soon this relationship is established and developed will vary with each individual woman and baby. Other factors, such as the views of the care-givers, also interfere with this process.

A number of studies (Klaus and Kennell, 1976; Ringler *et al.*, 1978) have shown that there are dynamic and complex behavioural cues involved in establishing this affinity and both partners play an important part in making the relationship either harmonious or dissonant. Macfarlane (1977) asserted that within four days of birth babies can follow a human face and recognize the voice and smell of a familiar person. Therefore, early contact with the mother is vital. It is the standard practice in maternity hospitals (including those in this study) to encourage the rooming-in method.

Rooming-in. This method allows the mother and baby to be kept together as a unit until they are discharged from hospital. The method has a number of advantages, for example, it provides a learning environment for the woman in which she is able to learn more quickly about her baby's needs. Another benefit is the stimulation she is able to give to her baby through cuddling, fondling, kissing and talking to him or her. The eye-to-eye contact is also of great importance since it is considered to evoke positive responses in the mother and women are continually searching for positive feedback from their baby.

It was observed that the women were not free to pick up and cuddle their baby and that those who did so were instructed by midwives to stop because of the risk of spoiling the child. This approach defeated the object of rooming-in and it caused anger, frustration and tension among the women who at times were eager to express their feelings towards their baby. Thus the woman's approach was guided by instinct while the midwives' was based largely on speculation. The concept of spoiling a newborn baby is debatable and possibly inappropriate at this early stage of developing a relationship.

In both hospitals the baby's cot was placed at the foot of the woman's bed; therefore, eye-to-eye contact between woman and baby was not possible. In one hospital, this method was used to facilitate easy access for staff between beds while in the other hospital, the emphasis was on keeping the ward tidy. After feeding their baby, the women would instinctively place the cot where the baby's face could be seen but the cot would be returned to the foot of the bed by the midwife. If a woman wanted to know the rationale behind the midwife's actions, she would be given one of the above reasons.

The new mother's needs. Both the midwives and the women shared the view that the motherhood role generates a variety of needs in its incumbent. However, there was a difference in emphasis placed on the priorities of those needs as illustrated in Table 9.1.

The difference in priority of needs as perceived by both groups was largely influenced by the perspective used to view motherhood. Thus the

Table 9.1 Midwives' and mothers' views of the mothers' needs following childbirth, listed according to priority

	Midwives' views of mothers' needs	*Mothers' views of mothers' needs*
1.	Maintenance of maternal physical health	Understanding the emotional needs of mothers
2.	Giving support (practical help with infant)	Teaching infant-orientated skills
3.	Giving information and advice	Information and advice
4.	Teaching infant-orientated skills	Supervision of skills
5.	Relaxed atmosphere	Relaxed atmosphere

Source: Compiled by the author.

midwives, using a biological and medical view of motherhood, considered the maintenance of maternal health to be of paramount importance. These women, however, viewed birth as a normal function, a view substantiated by the delivery of their baby via the normal route, with minimal trauma being sustained. Although they acknowledged the need for physical fitness, their focus of attention was on the emotional impact of childbirth. In the view of these women, midwives did not fully understand the mothers' emotional needs; consequently they perceived that their needs were not fully met by midwives.

Assessing the newly-delivered mother's needs. For the further development of the study it was necessary to find out how midwives assessed the needs of newly delivered mothers. The methods employed were observations of postnatal women, talking and listening to postnatal women, and using information contained in the woman's notes.

Many midwives stated that they assessed the needs of a newly delivered woman by observing the way she coped with her baby: if she coped 'adequately', her needs were considered to be minimal. Coping in this context referred to the woman's ability to feed and change her baby, as well as showing confidence in performing these activities. The woman's maternal interest in her baby, her level of confidence or fear of the baby were other cues that formed part of the observation assessment.

The data showed that the observations of women made by the midwives were irregular and inconsistent because midwifery care consisted of a series of tasks with no continuity of care. The women's medical records did not contain the depth of information to enable the midwife to make a full assessment of an individual woman's needs. The information from the daily ward reports on the woman's progress was brief and did not always mention the emotional aspects of care. Lastly, listening to and talking with women depended largely on how busy the wards were and the number of staff available.

For assessment and evaluation to be of benefit, all those concerned must be involved in the process. Thus, those engaged in the assessment and evaluation of maternal needs should take into account the woman's point of view, that is, how she sees her own needs. This exercise can be time-consuming and postnatal wards are often very busy and are not always suitably or adequately staffed. This raises the question of the importance placed on postnatal care by the midwifery managers who are responsible for allocating staff to the various areas of the maternity unit.

This section of the study showed that the care-givers (midwives) and the recipients (mothers) held different views of motherhood. This difference of views may be the cause of conflict, frustration and anger on the part of the recipients of care.

It is acknowledged that there may always be a difference in the way professionals (including midwives) and lay people interpret health, childbirth, and normally and abnormality (Freidson, 1970; McKinlay, 1972; Morgan *et al.*, 1985). However, in midwifery the difference could be narrowed by changes in the attitude of midwives with a movement towards midwife–client partnership in care, rather than the woman being expected to take on the role of patient with its associated behaviour. By definition, the role of client has a set of behaviour expectations different from that of the role of patient. The education of midwives should seek to broaden their knowledge and understanding of the concept of motherhood and encourage them to adopt a holistic approach to care, rather than to continue to see it primarily from a biological and medical perspective.

REFERENCES

Caplan, G. (1961) *An approach to community health.* Grune and Stratton, New York.

Comaroff, J. (1977) *Conflicting paradigms of pregnancy: Managing ambiguity in antenatal encounters.* In Davis, A. and Horobin, G. (eds), *Medical encounters: Experience of illness and treatment.* Croom Helm, London.

Denzin, N.K. (1970) *The research act: A theoretical introduction to sociological methods.* Aldine Publishing Company, Chicago.

Dyers, E.D. (1965) Parenthood as crisis – a re-study. *Marriage and Family Living, 25,* 196–201.

Fox, D.J. (1976) *Fundamentals of research in nursing.* Appleton Century Crofts, New York.

Freidson, E. (1970) *Professional dominance: The social structure of medical care.* Aldine Publishing Company, Chicago.

Freidson, E. (1975) *Profession of medicine: A study of the sociology of applied knowledge.* Harper & Row, New York.

Glaser, B.G. and Strauss, A. (1967) *The discovery of grounded theory: Strategies for qualitative research.* Aldine Publishing Company, Chicago.

Gold, R. (1958) Roles in sociological field observations. *Social Forces, 36* (March), 217–23.

Graham, H. and Oakley, A. (1981) Competing ideologies of reproduction: Medical and maternal perspectives on pregnancy. In Roberts, H. (ed.), *Women, health and reproduction,* Routledge and Kegan Paul, London.

Hart, N. (1977) Parenthood and patienthood: A dialectical autobiography. In Davis, A. and Horobin, G. (eds), *Medical encounters: Experience of illness and treatment,* Croom Helm, London.

Hobbs, D.E. (1965) Parenthood as crisis: A third study. *Journal of Marriage and Family, 27,* 367–72.

Junker, B. H. (1960) *Field work. An introduction to the social sciences.* University of Chicago Press, Chicago.

Klaus, H.M. and Kennell, J.H. (1976) *Maternal–infant interactions.* C.V. Mosby, St Louis.

Laryea, M.G.G. (1980) The midwives' role in the post-natal care of primiparae and their infants in the first 28 days following childbirth. Unpublished MPhil. thesis, Newcastle Polytechnic.

Le Masters, E.E. (1957) Parenthood as crisis. *Marriage and Family Living, 19,* 352–5.

Macfarlane, A. (1977) *The psychology of childbirth.* Open Books, London.

McKinlay, J.B. (1972) The sick role: Illness and pregnancy. *Social Science and*

Medicine, 6 (6), 561–72.

Morgan, M., Calnan, M. and Manning, N. (1985) *Sociological approaches to health and medicine.* Croom Helm, London.

Oakley, A. (1977) Cross cultural practices. In Chard, T. and Richards, M. (eds) *Benefits and hazards of the new obstetrics: Clinics in developmental medicine,* no. 64. William Heinemann Medical Books, London.

Raphael, D. (1975) *Being female. Reproduction, power and change.* Moulton Publishers, The Hague.

Rapoport, R. (1963) Normal crises: Family structure and mental health. *Family Process, 2* (1), 68–80.

Reeder, S.R., Mastroianni, L., Martin, L.L. and Fitzpatrick, E. (1971) *Maternity nursing,* 12th edn. Lippincott, Philadelphia.

Ringler, R., Trause, M.A., Klaus, M. and Kennell, J. (1978) The effect of extra post-partum contacts and maternal speech patterns on children's IQs, speech and language comprehension at five. *Child Development, 49,* 862–65.

Romalis, S. (1985) Struggle between providers and recipients: The case of birth practice. In Lewin, E. and Olesen, V. (eds), *Women, health and healing: Towards a new perspective,* Tavistock, New York.

Rossi, A. (1974) Transition to parenthood. In Greenblat, C. (ed.), *The marriage game,* Random House, New York.

Selltiz, C., Jahoda, M., Deutsch, M. and Cook, S. W. (1966) *Research methods in social relations,* 3rd edn. Holt, Rinehart & Winston, New York.

Stacey, M. (1969) *Methods of social research.* Pergamon Press, Oxford.

Strauss, A.L. (1962) Transformation of identity. In Rose, A. (ed.), *Behaviour and social processes: An interactionist approach,* Houghton Mifflin Company, New York.

CHAPTER TEN

Models of childbirth and social class: a study of 80 working-class primigravidae

James McIntosh

INTRODUCTION

The distinction between 'natural' and medical models of childbirth has been a common theme in the sociological literature on reproduction (Comaroff, 1977; Nash and Nash, 1979; Graham and Oakley, 1981; Macintyre, 1981; Nelson, 1983; Oakley, 1984b). Whereas the medical model is said to view the event as inherently problematic, requiring medical intervention and control in order to be accomplished successfully, the natural model regards it as a normal biological process over which the women themselves should exert active control and in which medical intervention should be undertaken only in exceptional circumstances. These two models, in turn, imply very different measures of success. With the medical model, success is measured in accordance with narrowly defined medical criteria, whereas with the natural model, success is assessed in holistic terms. From the perspective of the natural approach, a 'successful' birth is one that is accomplished without the assistance of drugs or other forms of intervention and in which the woman herself has retained control over the process.

Advocates of natural childbirth have, in various guises, been a powerful voice in the maternity arena in recent years. Their major criticism of the contemporary management of childbirth has concerned the increasing medicalization of the process (Arms, 1975; Haire, 1978). Modern obstetric practice is said to have harmful iatrogenic consequences as well as being emotionally unsatisfactory for women. In addition, it is claimed that women themselves are increasingly opposed to the medicalization of labour and delivery and seek a form of childbirth that is more 'natural' in the sense of being accomplished without the assistance of artificial means of pain relief and other forms of intervention. In recent years, a number of studies have helped to reinforce this view by providing evidence of a considerable amount of dissatisfaction with the medical management of pregnancy and childbirth (Topliss, 1970; Oakley, 1975; Kitzinger, 1978;

Blehar, 1979; Cartwright, 1979; Graham and Oakley, 1981). This dis-satisfaction has centred upon a dislike of interventions – such as the induction of labour or episiotomy – complaints about the quality of human relations in maternity care, and a desire to be in control of the birth process. Many women also object to the customary preparation for childbirth, which includes an enema and the removal of pubic hair. Some authors have claimed that all of this amounts to a widespread rejection of the medical management of childbirth.

However, there is evidence to suggest that the orientation towards childbirth represented above is by no means universal. Specifically, there would appear to be considerable social class differences in women's atti-tudes towards childbirth and its management. Working-class women, it would seem, are less opposed to medical intervention and control and less likely to espouse the cause of natural childbirth (Reid, 1983; Reid, Gutteridge and McIlwaine, 1983; Nelson, 1983). This chapter seeks to augment our knowledge of these differences by reporting on a study of the expectations, experiences and reactions to childbirth of a sample of 80 working-class primigravidae.

SAMPLE AND METHODS

The data presented in this chapter were collected in 1982 in the course of a larger prospective study of first-time mothers. Initially 80 women were selected randomly from three Glasgow antenatal clinics. However, due to sample wastage, this number had declined to 68 by the time of the first postnatal interview. The sample was exclusively working class with approximately half of the women coming from social class 3b (37) and the other half (43) from social classes 4 and 5. Roughly half of the women (42) were aged 20 years or under at first contact and just under one quarter (18) were single parents. A further 19 pregnancies were pre-nuptial conceptions. Unemployment levels were high with 29% (18 of 62) of partners and 28% of single parents (5 of 18) being unemployed at the beginning of the study. In short, then, the sample was broadly representative of working-class primiparae as a whole.

Contact with the subjects extended from the seventh month of pregnancy until the child was about nine months old. Each woman was interviewed on six occasions – once prenatally around the seventh month and five times during the postnatal phase – with the first postnatal inter-view being administered at one month postpartum. The interviews were semi-structured and combined fixed questions with a flexible repertoire of topics that were explored in a more open-ended way. All interviews were conducted in the subjects' own homes and were tape-recorded. Information on objective features of the women's confinements was obtained from their case records.

Some of the data are based upon responses to structured questions. These were coded and analysed in the usual way and this chapter is largely concerned with the presentation of these findings. However, in order to gain further insight into the processes we were examining, we also employed a number of open-ended questions which allowed a more exploratory and spontaneous set of discussions about our sample's attitudes towards childbirth. This qualitative approach enabled us to investigate topics raised by the respondents themselves and to explore them in ways that were relevant to the experiences and orientations of particular individuals. In this way we were able to consider emergent themes that were not covered by our fixed questions. At the end of the study, the interview transcripts were reviewed in order to identify the topics or themes contained in these open-ended responses and the contexts in which statements were made. These topics were subsequently categorized, coded and analysed. This method has the advantage that analytical categories are derived from the data themselves rather than being predetermined. Since these qualitative data were not obtained in a controlled way, we would obviously make no claims as to their representativeness. The value of this approach lies not in its quantitative contribution but in the way in which it enhances the interpretation of more rigid quantitative data and so improves insights into the context and determinants of particular kinds of behaviour. It is upon data assembled in this manner that our qualitative comments are based.

FINDINGS

Prenatal attitudes towards the birth

Expectations and their sources. In the course of the antenatal interview, we asked our respondents what they thought the birth would be like and generally explored their attitudes towards it. On the basis of their replies, we defined our sample as being either positive or negative in their expectations. Those respondents who said that they were looking forward to the birth in some way or who referred to potentially rewarding or fulfilling aspects of the experience were classed as being positive in their orientation towards it. Those, on the other hand, whose expectations were entirely concerned with the anxiety-provoking aspects of childbirth were classed as negative. Three women held positive and negative views simultaneously, and were defined as having mixed expectations. Nine respondents were classified as being neutral in orientation in the sense that, while they expressed no worries or fears in relation to the birth, they did not, on the other hand, appear to regard it at all positively.

As Table 10.1 reveals, our sample's expectations of the birth were almost overwhelmingly negative. Only 6 out of the 80 women (i.e. those in the 'positive' and 'mixed' categories) expressed any positive feelings towards it, although some of those who did were clearly very much looking forward to the experience:

> I'm just terribly excited. It's like gettin' a Christmas present. I'm no' worried about anything. Ah just think it'll be great.

Table 10.1 Women's expectations of childbirth

Expectations	no.	%
Positive	3	4
Negative	62	77
Neutral	9	11
Mixed	3	4
Don't know	3	4
Total	80	100

Source: Compiled by the author.

Ah think it'll be terrific. Ah'm not frightened in the least. Ah'm lookin' forward to it that much ah can hardly wait.

However, the expectations of the great majority of our sample (77%) were negative. They did not view the prospect of childbirth as being in any way a potentially positive experience. For them, the birth was simply a hurdle to be surmounted on the way to motherhood. Their main sentiment was a sense of fear and foreboding, a major aspect of which was a fear of the unknown (Macintyre, 1981; Nelson, 1983):

Ah'm scared. Ah don't know what it's going to be like. Ah just can't put myself in that position. Ah sit at night and wonder ... That's what frightens me: this fear o' the unknown. Ye know, not knowing what it's gonnae be like.

Twelve women described themselves as being 'terrified' at the prospect of the birth and many others were clearly just as frightened. For example, one respondent confessed:

Ah'm very scared. Ah can't stand pain and everybody tells me it's really sore especially when the head's coming out. Sometimes ah sit at night and greet [cry] ah'm that scared.

Not surprisingly, perhaps, the biggest source of fear was the prospect of pain during labour and delivery. Other anxieties included having a caesarean section, having forceps or having an episiotomy. Sixteen women were also concerned about how they would recognize that they were in labour. Another major apprehension related to the actual delivery itself, with 14 women spontaneously expressing concern over their ability to expel the baby through what was, to them, a relatively narrow opening:

What really worries me is gettin' the baby out. Y'know, the actual delivery of it. A baby's such a big thing.

Table 10.2 Sources of information about childbirth ($n = 80$)*

Friends	36
Sister	21
Mother	19
Other relatives	18
Books, etc.	18
Other lay sources	14
Television	7
Professional sources	4
None	7

Source: Compiled by the author.
*Most respondents reported more than one source.

Our sample's fears were largely based upon the accounts of childbirth that they received from friends and relatives. As Table 10.2 shows, lay sources predominated when it came to information about the birth. Professional sources, the media and other reading materials were much less prominent. Although the accounts of childbirth which these women received from their lay networks ranged from the horrific to 'it's as easy as shelling peas', the great majority of these descriptions were alarming. Overall, the effect of information from lay sources was to promote and reinforce a negative perception of childbirth. Many friends and relatives appeared to almost delight in recounting the more gruesome aspects of their own experiences or those of their acquaintances. Certainly, for our sample, accounts of childbirth that provoked alarm were considerably more common than those that provided reassurance. Our respondents sought to cope with these negative messages by stressing individual differences and the uniqueness of each individual's experience. They reassured themselves that everyone is different and that, while birth might be a traumatic experience for some, this would not necessarily be so in their case:

> Ah'm a bit scared but ah hope ah'll be alright when it comes to it. Ah just feel that everybody's different. You shouldn't listen to anybody that tells you whit it's gonnae be like 'cause you're gonnae be different.

> Ah get scared when folk tell me the terrible times that they've had. But ah just go, 'That'll no' happen tae me, ah'm different.' Ye see ah think everybody's different ... no two births are the same.

So, the great majority of our sample viewed their forthcoming childbirth as a frightening and unpredictable experience.

Interestingly, there were no social class differences to this, with social class 3 women being just as negative as those from social classes 4 and 5.

Given their apprehensions, the major concern of our sample was not with positive aspects of childbirth or with deriving a sense of fulfilment from the experience. Rather, their concern was with how to retain their composure and avoid the embarassment of breaking down or losing control during the ordeal that they anticipated childbirth would be. In fact, for some, coping appeared to be almost more important than what they had to cope with. These feelings were keenly expressed by one respondent in the following way:

> Ah just hope ah don't get too excited or lose the head. Ye don't know how yer gonnae be 'til ye've done it. Ah might completely freak out and disgrace myself.

This set of priorities was reflected in our subjects' attitudes towards pain relief and intervention. Only three of our respondents indicated any desire for what could be termed a 'natural' childbirth. For them the experience of pain was an essential part of the experience of giving birth: without it you could not claim to know what it was 'really' like to have a baby:

> Ah'd like it to be natural, y'know, so that ah can say, 'Ah've had a baby.' Ah don't really want the pain but ah think if ah had a choice ah'd rather do without the drugs and just have it naturally.

> Ah'd rather have it without anything. If you didn't feel it, you'd feel you were missin' out, y'know. Ye widnae really know what it was like tae have a baby!

However, the great majority of our sample had no wish whatsoever to experience the birth in its entirety. They were simply concerned to get it over with as quickly as possible and with as little pain as possible. The following extracts are fairly typical of this group:

> Ah've no wish tae experience the birth. Ah'll just be glad when it's all over with. . . . Ah just want tae have ma baby. What I'd like is tae get put tae sleep and not know whit's happening.

> Gie me a jag [injection] an' knock me out an' waken me up when the baby's there and that'll be just fine.

Attitudes towards pain relief. Consistent with this philosophy, two-thirds of our sample expressed a positive desire for some form of pain relief during labour when we questioned them antenatally (Table 10.3). Only one in six said that they did not want any although a quarter of the women had not formed an opinion at that stage. Among those who said they did not want pain relief, about half said it was because they were afraid of injections and two felt that analgesia might affect the baby. The other reason given for not wanting pain relief was a desire to have the baby as 'naturally' as possible. Women giving this as a reason came exclusively from the ranks of those with a positive or neutral attitude towards the birth. These women believed that the introduction of pain

Table 10.3 Pain relief preferences

Preferences	no.	%
Wanted some	49	61
Wanted none	13	16
Don't know	18	23
Total	80	100

Source: Compiled by the author.

relief would deprive them of a major part of the experience of giving birth.

We also asked those respondents who said they wanted pain relief which form they would prefer. The preferences which they gave must, of course, have reflected the women's knowledge of different forms of pain relief at that time and should not, therefore, be regarded as representing fully informed choices. Having said that, the most popular method by far was the epidural; its main advantage, from the women's point of view, being that it eliminated all sensation of pain (Table 10.4). 'Gas and air' was second in popularity while only a handful mentioned pethidine. Some women had no particular preference and were prepared to accept anything that eliminated the pain. As one said, 'Ah think ah'd just take anything if it was sore.' In common with their information on childbirth generally, our sample's knowledge of pain relief was, at this stage, derived almost entirely from family and friends.

The prospect of intervention. Now, while the prospect of pain relief tended to be positively welcomed by our sample, their attitude towards intervention was much more one of acceptance. In short, intervention was tolerated as an inevitable part of the process of giving birth and regarded, at worst, as a necessary evil. Many viewed it philosophically:

It would be nice to have it without any artificial things but, if it needs it, it needs it.

This orientation is perhaps best illustrated by our sample's attitudes towards induction of labour. We first asked them if they had heard about induction or the fact that women's labours could be started artificially. Just over two-thirds of them (67%) said that they had. We then went on to ask those who professed knowledge of induction what they would feel about their labour being induced. We see from Table 10.5 that while about one-quarter of our respondents raised objections to their labour being induced, the majority either expressed unqualified acceptance of it – for example, 'You've no option if you're overdue' – or said that they

Table 10.4 Type of pain relief preferred

Pain relief	no.	%
Epidural	22	45
'Entonox'	9	18
Pethidine	3	6
Don't know	15	31
Total	49	100

Source: Compiled by the author.

Table 10.5 Attitudes towards induction of labour

Attitudes*	no.	%
Negative feelings	15	28
Acceptance	24	44
Positive feelings	0	0
Depends	6	11
Don't know	9	17
Total	54	100

Source: Compiled by the author.

*Responses in answer to the survey question, 'What would you feel about being induced?'

would accept it as long as it was being done for a 'good' reason: that is, for reasons other than those of convenience. None of the women regarded labour being induced as something that they would welcome.

These, then, were some of the main features of our sample's expectations of the birth and their attitudes towards it. Before their reactions to the birth itself are described, some of the main objective features of their confinements are briefly outlined.

Content of the birth

Table 10.6 shows the proportion of our sample having different forms of delivery. About half (47%) had an unassisted vaginal delivery, 35% required forceps, and 12 women had a caesarean section, 8 of which were emergencies. Although not shown in this Table, episiotomy was almost universal, being carried out in 90% of cases. Excluding the four elective

Table 10.6 Mode of delivery

Delivery	no.	%
Normal	32	47
Forceps	24	35
Caesarean section (elective)	4	6
Caesarean section (emergency)	8	12
Total	68	100

Source: Compiled by the author.

caesarean sections, 38 of the remaining 64 labours (59%) were spontaneous in onset; the rest (41%) were induced (Table 10.7). In addition, however, 20 of the spontaneous labours were also augmented. This means that only 18 of the 64 births (28%) had no intervention to influence either the onset or pace of labour. These figures compare with similar rates for the induction and acceleration of labour reported elsewhere at the time of the study (Cartwright, 1979; Macintyre, 1981).

The great majority of our sample had some form of pain relief during labour. In fact, excluding the 12 who had a caesarean section, only three out of the remaining 56 women received no pain relief. Of those who did get something, 32 (60%) had pethidine and about half (26) had an epidural. Some, of course, had both. Ten of the women who had a caesarean section also received epidural analgesia, so that the total proportion of our sample having an epidural was 53%.

Reactions to the birth

This section documents the ways in which our sample perceived and reacted to the birth. It is difficult to summarize the diverse range of experiences and reactions contained in our sample's accounts of their childbirth. Each woman had her own unique story to tell and every account provided fresh insight into the process of giving birth. For example, some births had apparently been relatively easy:

It's just like doin' the toilet, only bigger. It was no bother.

Ah thoroughly enjoyed every bit of it. Ah don't know what all the fuss is about.

Others had obviously been extremely unpleasant:

It was a terrible experience. One o' the worst o' my life. It seemed tae go on for months. Ah thought it wis never going to end.

I had everything. I was induced, then they kept speeding up and

Table 10.7 Onset of labour ($n = 64$)

Onset of labour	no.	%
Spontaneous	38	59
Accelerated	20	31
Induced	26	41

Source: Compiled by the author.

Table excludes 4 elective caesarean sections.

slowing down the contractions and I had an epidural and forceps and an episiotomy. And through it all they didnae tell ye anything. It wis terrible. I felt like a lump of mince.

It is clearly impossible to retain the full flavour, richness and variety of the women's experiences in the present context. Instead, certain selected aspects of our sample's experiences and reactions are described.

Mother's 'satisfaction' with the birth. As a number of authors have pointed out, the concept of consumer satisfaction can be highly problematic (Riley, 1977; Cartwright, 1979; Porter and Macintyre, 1984; Lumley, 1985). In particular, the meaning and status of replies to questions relating to individuals' satisfaction with particular services is difficult to assess. For example, consumers frequently assume that the existing system or practice must be well-founded and therefore the best that can be provided. Alongside this they commonly lack the awareness or experience of alternatives against which current services could be measured. This means that expressions of satisfaction often have more to do with low expectations than any positive feelings towards the service in question. The concept of 'satisfaction' also tends to be too general to be useful as a category for summarizing consumer reactions and, as such, frequently begs as many questions as it answers. All this means that to have simply asked the women whether or not they were 'satisfied' with the birth and the way in which it had been managed would have produced replies that would have been relatively meaningless.

Having said that, however, we did also believe that it was important, for analytical purposes, to formulate some sort of summary statement of the extent to which the women's experiences could be described as positive or negative. Accordingly, we constructed a composite category of 'satisfaction' on the basis of the women's replies to a series of questions concerning how the birth had gone, whether there were any things about it they had not liked, whether they would have liked anything to have been done differently or not done at all and so on. Their replies were then scrutinized for complaints: that is, things that women felt could and should have been done differently. We then defined as 'dissatisfied' all of those who reported one or more complaints about the conduct of the birth. Using this criterion, we found that the great majority of our sample (74%) were satisfied with the way in which their labour and delivery had been conducted (Table 10.8). Only one-quarter of the women raised objections of any kind. We found no correlation between satisfaction and the age and social class of the woman or her attendance at preparation classes.

Correspondence between expectations and experiences. In addition to assessing our sample's 'satisfaction' with the birth, we also attempted to measure the extent to which their expectations had been met. It will be recalled that the majority of our respondents had negative expectations of childbirth. However, when we asked them afterwards if the experience had been better or worse than they had expected, the majority (53%) replied that it had been better (Table 10.9). Less than a quarter of our sample had found the experience to be worse than expected. Fifteen said it had been mixed: that is, some parts of the birth had been better than expected and others had been worse. Two said the experience had been as expected. We found no association between our respondents' assessments of the birth and their age, social class or attendance at birth preparation classes.

Table 10.8 Satisfaction with the birth

Women's reported feelings	no.	%
Satisfied	50	74
Dissatisfied	18	26
Total	68	100

Source: Compiled by the author.

Table 10.9 Women's assessments of the birth

Assessments	no.	%
Better than expected	36	53
Worse than expected	15	22
Mixed	15	22
As expected	2	3
Total	68	100

Source: Compiled by the author.

It was clear from supplementary questioning that whether the birth was assessed as better or worse than expected depended upon the duration of labour, the amount of pain experienced and the extent to which the woman believed she had been able to remain in control of her emotions and behaviour. For example:

> I'd listened tae a lot o' people saying, 'Oh, it's terrible' and that. But ah never really took it in. It's just as well 'cause it was much worse than I thought it'd be. It was much sorer and it went on for ages. Ah thought it was never goin' tae end.

> It wis worse than I expected. I really cracked up and was shoutin' and screamin'. I feel embarassed thinking about it. I didnae think it would get me like that.

In other words, 'better' births were shorter and less painful than anticipated and had not led to the woman losing control of herself. Although it was not mentioned by the women themselves, it is also possible that the fact that they had been able to cope with an experience that they feared they might not be able to handle might have contributed to the high proportion of women who felt the birth had been better than expected.

Future intentions. In a further attempt to investigate our respondents' reactions to the birth, we asked them what they would like the birth of their next baby – assuming they had one – to be like and, in particular, whether there were any ways in which they would like it to differ from their recent experience. We were particularly interested here in the proportion of women expressing a desire for an intervention-free birth.

In fact, only six women indicated that they would prefer a 'natural' birth – in the sense of having no pain relief or other forms of intervention – on a future occasion. It is also interesting to note that only one of the three women who had originally expressed a preference for a natural birth wanted one next time, the other two had found pain relief in particular to be indispensable. On the other hand, though, five women who had indicated no desire for a natural birth originally said that they wanted one next time. This change of heart was largely a result of negative experiences of intervention and a consequent desire to avoid it in the future. However, this decision was also buttressed by the confidence that the women had gained as a result of having gone through the process. Much of the original uncertainty and fear of the unknown had gone. Childbirth was now a known entity and they felt that, in future, they could cope on their own.

Reactions to pain relief. Thus, the majority of the respondents appeared to be satisfied with their first experience of childbirth. For most of them, the discomfort involved and the interventions that were undertaken were either simply accepted as an inevitable and unavoidable part of the process or, in the case of some procedures, actually welcomed. This applied to pain relief in particular.

At the first postnatal interview we asked our sample what they thought of the pain relief they had received and whether they would have it again. Three-quarters of the women (77%) reacted positively to pain relief and only one in six expressed a negative view and said that they had not liked it or would rather not have had it. (Table 10.10). The principal benefit of pain relief from the women's point of view was that it addressed their main concerns in relation to the birth: that is, it reduced or removed the experience of pain and thereby greatly assisted their ability to cope with the experience and maintain composure and self-control.

For most women, then, pain relief was very much welcomed. In fact, many volunteered the view that they did not think they could have coped without it. The epidural proved to be particularly popular with our sample, its main advantage being that it completely eliminated pain, while at the same time, it had none of the adverse effects upon the women's consciousness that were often associated with 'gas and air' or pethidine. Over 80% of those who had an epidural (21 out of 26) said that they would have it again.

However, there was a negative side to pain relief as well. Some women complained that the pethidine they received had not worked, while others claimed that it worked too well and had made them so 'dopey' that, in some cases, they were not fully conscious at the birth:

> See that pethidine, it knocked me out. There's a lot o' things ah can't remember because o' that drug.... They kept havin' tae wake me up sayin', "Come on, he can't wait." I'd keep wakening up and sayin', "Isn't it finished now?" and they kept sayin' "No". And ah felt another needle goin' intae me and that was me out again. He wis born wi' forceps.

Epidural analgesia tended to excite the most extreme reactions from the respondents. While it was the form of pain relief which elicited the

Table 10.10 Reactions to pain relief received

Reactions to analgesia	no.	%
Positive	41	77
Negative	9	17
Mixed	3	6
Total	53	100

Source: Compiled by the author.

Table excludes reactions of those who had a caesarean section.

most favourable responses, it also had the distinction of provoking the most critical comments. Eight women claimed that their epidural had not been entirely successful or complained of after-effects. Two women said they regretted having it because it meant missing out on an important part of the experience of giving birth.

Finally, five women complained of feeling pressurized into having pain relief. It was not that deliberate pressure was put on them. What appeared to happen was that repeated offers of pain relief were interpreted by women as implying that the staff wanted them to take something. It was a perceived pressure that some found difficult to resist:

> I felt forced intae having the epidural. They [staff] kept coming and asking if ah wanted something. They said, "If your pains are sore, you're better wi' something." Ah mean they try tae push ye intae having something. So I agreed.

Acceleration of labour. Just as pain relief was welcomed by the majority of the women, so too was the acceleration of labour viewed positively by most of them. In fact, apart from the fact that only one woman actually complained about her labour being speeded up, the majority of women (81%) indicated that they welcomed the fact that their labour had been accelerated. The explanation for the popularity of this procedure may be that it has the advantage of shortening labour while, at the same time, any negative effects in the form of additional pain are largely counteracted by pain relief. For some women, getting the birth over quickly was a more important consideration than the level of discomfort experienced and four claimed that they would prefer a shorter, accelerated labour even if it meant an increase in pain.

Sources of dissatisfaction. While the majority of our sample appeared to be satisfied with the birth, a proportion of them were not. The major source of dissatisfaction for these women was the amount and type of intervention to which they were subjected. This was reflected in a fairly strong relationship between intervention and our various measures of satisfaction. Induction of labour was particularly unpopular with the women, with almost all of those who experienced it saying that they disliked it. The artificial rupturing of their membranes was especially unpopular as a method of starting labour, with the women often regarding it almost as a sort of violation. Our respondents' view of induction was clearly very different from their attitude towards the acceleration of labour. In contrast to the latter, induction was regarded as, at best, a necessary evil that involved considerable discomfort and conferred few obvious benefits. These attitudes are entirely consistent with Cartwright's (1979) finding that 78% of women whose labour was induced would not want an induction again.

Not surprisingly, those women whose labour had been induced were more likely to express dissatisfaction with the birth and to say that it had been worse than expected (Table 10.11). Fewer than half (45%) of those

Table 10.11 Relationship between induction of labour and women's assessments of the birth

| | Satisfaction with the birth | | | | Assessment of the birth in terms of expectations | | | | | | | | |
| | Satisfied | | Dissatisfied | | Better | | Worse | | Mixed | | As expected | |
	no.	%	no.	%	no.	%	no.	%	no.	%	no.	%
Induced	15	58	11	42	10	45	6	27	6	27	0	0
Not induced	31	84	6	16	21	62	4	12	8	24	1	3

Source: Compiled by the author.

whose labour had been induced had found the birth to be better than expected, as opposed to nearly two-thirds (62%) of those whose labour was not induced. Similarly, whereas 84% of those not induced were 'satisfied' with the birth, the corresponding figure for the induced group was 58%.

There was also a strong correlation between women's assessments of the birth and the use of forceps (Table 10.12). In short, women whose delivery was forceps-assisted were considerably less likely to report that the birth had been better than expected. Only one-third of those having forceps said that it had been better, as opposed to two-thirds of those who did not have forceps. Of course the reason for this association may have less to do with the use of forceps per se than with the fact that their use is indicative of a birth that is 'bad' or problematic in other ways.

The other major source of dissatisfaction for these women concerned an alleged lack of explanation of what was happening and being done to them during labour and delivery. We asked our sample whether the various interventions had been explained to them. In many instances it would appear that they had not (Table 10.13). While it would seem that induction of labour was nearly always explained, the same could not be

Table 10.12 The use of forceps and women's assessments of the birth

	Better		*Worse*		*Mixed*		*As expected*		*Total*
	no.	*%*	*no.*	*%*	*no.*	*%*	*no.*	*%*	
Forceps	9	37	4	17	10	42	1	4	24
No forceps	22	69	6	19	4	12	0	0	32

Source: Compiled by the author.

Table 10.13 Was intervention explained?

Intervention	*No. explained*	*No. unexplained*	*No. with no recollection*
Induction	25	0	1
Acceleration of labour	14	6	0
Forceps	18	6	0
Epidural	21	3	2
Pethidine	21	5	6
Episiotomy	16	30	4

Source: Compiled by the author.

said for the acceleration of labour or the use of forceps, both of which were apparently unexplained in about one-quarter of cases. As we can see from Table 10.13, pain relief was not always explained, with three women claiming that even the epidural had not been explained to them. Two-thirds of the women reported that their episiotomy had not been explained. The following quotation was fairly typical of the latter:

> It wis after the baby was born they told me. They said, "We had to cut you." Y'know, they never told me when they cut me that they were cuttin' me. And ah never felt it. It was only after when they said, "You'll need to have stitches," that ah said, "Whit for?"

Now, all of this needs to be qualified since at the time that most of these procedures were being carried out, the women were probably not at their most receptive. By their own admission, many felt doped, confused, exhausted or distracted during confinement. It is therefore entirely possible that, in a proportion of cases, explanation had in fact been given but had simply not registered. Nevertheless, whether it was real or imagined, a perceived lack of explanation created a lot of anxiety and was a major source of complaint for our respondents. The following quotations are typical of their comments:

> They should tell you a lot more aboot what's goin' on. You're kept in the dark all the time and ye just worry and imagine things. Yer imagination runs away wi' you and ye think o' the worst.

> Ah don't think they explain enough to you. Ah mean, ah know it's a sort o' everyday occurrence to them but they don't seem to understand how nervous you are. You think to yourself, "Oh God, something's happening to me," and you're scared but they don't explain what's going on.

Finally, five women complained of a lack of continuity in the staff who attended them. For example:

> I think more than anything you had too many different people doing things to you.... Obviously if you're going for a long time it's got to be different doctors and nurses but you were just getting to know a face, gaining confidence in that person when you got somebody else.

Overall, though, our sample's attitudes towards the staff who attended them were favourable. Insofar as the women had complaints about the birth, these related to intervention rather than to human relations aspects of their care.

Adverse emotional outcomes. These, then, were some of the ways in which our sample reacted to the experience of childbirth. Clearly, the content and management of labour and delivery had strong implications for the women's subjective reactions to the birth and their degree of satisfaction with it. The amount and type of medical intervention and the perceived adequacy of communication were found to be particularly important in producing negative assessments.

However, while our sample's subjective reactions to childbirth clearly constitute an important measure of outcome, we also considered that it was important to establish whether their experiences had any more objective significance, specifically in terms of their effect upon the emotional health of the women. There was already evidence from elsewhere of an apparent connection between the experience of childbirth and certain adverse emotional outcomes. For example, Oakley (1980) had found the amount of intervention that a woman was subjected to and her overall satisfaction with the birth to be predictive of both postnatal blues and postnatal depression. We therefore investigated whether a similar pattern was obtained in our own sample.

Firstly, we examined our data for a possible relationship between the occurrence of postnatal blues and measures such as the women's satisfaction with the birth and the amount and type of intervention that was carried out. We defined postnatal blues as the experience of depressed mood at any time during the first week postpartum. However, since a tendency to cry in the immediate postnatal period is frequently used as a defining characteristic of the blues, we also distinguished between those women whose depressed mood was accompanied by crying and those for whom it was not. In neither case did we find any association between the blues and the various measures that we selected for comparison (McIntosh, 1986). No correlation was found with individual types of intervention. Nor did we find any relationship with the amount of intervention undertaken. A birth intervention score was calculated for each woman based upon the number of intervention procedures that were carried out. These included induction of labour, the acceleration of labour, forceps delivery, epidural analgesia, episiotomy and the administration of other pain-relieving drugs excluding gas and air. Each procedure was assigned a value of one, giving a maximum potential score of six for each woman. As Table 10.14 shows, there was no correlation between these intervention scores and the occurrence of the blues. Finally, we found no association between postnatal blues and the women's satisfaction with the birth (as defined earlier) or whether it had been better or worse than expected.

We also investigated whether there was any relationship between our respondents' experience of childbirth and the occurrence of depression in the postnatal phase. We defined as 'depressed' all women who experienced depressed mood for a period of at least 14 days at any stage after the first postpartum week. Using this definition, we found that two-thirds of our sample (38 out of 60) experienced depression at some time during the nine months following the birth of their baby. However, we found no significant correlation between depression and any of the birth-related factors that we selected for analysis. For example, no individual item of intervention – including the induction and acceleration of labour, epidural anaesthesia and forceps delivery – was found to be predictive of depression. However, although individual procedures were not predictive of depression, we did detect a tendency for its incidence to rise with increasing amounts of intervention. Table 10.15 reveals that while only 50% (12 of 24) of those with three or fewer interventions became depressed, 77% (20 of 26) of those with four or more did so. However, while suggestive of a trend in a particular direction, these findings did not reach statistical significance. We also found no association between depression and subjective features of the birth such as the women's satisfaction with the event and the extent to which their expectations had been met (Tables 10.16 and 10.17). Instead, depression was found to be associated with non-birth factors such as the pressures and demands of motherhood and aspects of social and economic disadvantage (McIntosh, 1985).

Table 10.14 Postnatal blues and the amount of intervention during labour and delivery

Number of interventions	Postnatal blues no.	No postnatal blues no.
1	3	1
2	9	2
3	9	4
4	13	6
5	5	4
Total	39	17

Source: Compiled by the author.

Table 10.15 Postnatal depression and birth intervention score

Intervention score	Depressed no.	Not depressed no.
1	2	1
2	5	6
3	5	5
4	14	3
5	6	3
Total	32	18

Source: Compiled by the author.

Table 10.16 Satisfaction with the birth and postnatal depression

Satisfaction	Depressed no.	Not depressed no.
Satisfied	29	15
Dissatisfied	9	6
Total	38	21

Source: Compiled by the author.

Table 10.17 Postnatal depression and women's assessments of the birth

Assessment of the birth	Depressed no.	Not depressed no.
Better than expected	19	9
Worse than expected	8	5
Mixed	9	6
Total	36	20

Source: Compiled by the author.

DISCUSSION

Our working-class sample's expectations of childbirth were largely negative and utilitarian. Although a small number of women viewed childbirth as a positive and potentially rewarding experience, the great majority regarded it as an ordeal and as a means to an end rather than as an end in itself. There was little support among our sample for what could be termed a 'natural' birth. As one 20-year-old commented, 'I couldn't have cared less what they did to me. I was just wanting it all finished.' Our respondents' priorities were to get the birth over with as quickly as possible, to keep pain and discomfort to a minimum, and to maintain self-control during what they anticipated would be a frightening and unpredictable experience. Given these priorities, pain relief and the acceleration of labour were generally welcomed. Alongside this, there was a general acceptance of the medicalization of childbirth although, as shown, there was discontent with certain aspects of intervention and with an alleged lack of explanation. In general, though, intervention was not regarded as intrinsically bad and, at worst, tended to be accepted as a necessary evil.

Overall, our respondents appeared to be relatively satisfied with their experiences of childbirth. Most said that it had been better than they had anticipated and only a minority voiced complaints about its conduct. Where negative feelings were expressed, they were found to be closely related to the content of labour and delivery and the way in which these had been managed. The birth as a whole was assessed in terms of how long it lasted, the amount of pain experienced, and the extent to which the woman felt she had been able to control her reactions. Forms of intervention that facilitated the achievement of these objectives were generally welcomed even if they themselves involved a measure of discomfort.

Insofar as it is possible to make comparisons, our sample's satisfaction with the birth appeared to exceed that described in some of the literature. For example, whereas 47% of Oakley's (1979) mainly middle-class sample reported that the experience had been worse than they expected, only 22% of our respondents did so. However, the levels of satisfaction expressed by our sample do not necessarily represent preferences in any absolute sense and certainly should not be taken to indicate that their experiences of childbirth were either positive or trouble-free. In fact, our sample's relatively favourable reactions to the birth are more likely to have been a product of their particular expectations and priorities than the result of any sense of positive satisfaction with the event (Riley, 1977). In short, it is probable that our sample of working-class women were less critical of their experience of childbirth because they expected less of it. However, our sample's expectations are themselves likely to have been partly conditioned by their awareness of alternative approaches to childbirth and their perceptions of their feasibility. Here our evidence suggests that our respondents had been socialized or schooled in a passive approach to childbirth and in an acceptance of the medicalization of labour and delivery. Certainly, they appeared to be unaware of any possibility of challenging the traditional medical management of childbirth or of expressing their own preferences. Similarly, they displayed little awareness of 'natural' approaches to giving birth. We know from other work that, when unaware of alternatives, women tend to accept the service that they are given in the assumption that the prevailing system must be best (Riley, 1977; Cartwright, 1979; Porter and Macintyre, 1984). On the basis of this, it could be argued that the women in our study accepted the medicalization of childbirth not because they preferred it but because they were unaware that they had a choice. However, even where this awareness did exist, alternative approaches tended to be rejected because the women lacked confidence in their ability to cope with them, this having been effectively undermined by the welter of negative accounts that they received from almost every source.

Our sample's low expectations and utilitarian approach to childbirth may also account for the fact that, in contrast with certain other studies (e.g., Pitt, 1968; Oakley, 1980), we found no association between the women's experiences and objective outcomes such as postnatal blues and depression. After all, it is not birth-related events themselves that are important in producing adverse emotional outcomes but the way in which they are perceived and interpreted. These interpretations will, in turn, be heavily influenced by the sorts of expectations that women bring to the experience. Given the particular priorities of the women in our study, intervention and the medicalization of childbirth generally were probably much less likely to provoke feelings of failure or disappointment than might be the case for groups who place a higher value on the birth experience itself. If this analysis is correct, it means that the effects of intervention during labour and delivery are relative and not absolute, since they depend entirely upon the way in which individual women perceive and interpret them. In this way, birth experiences may have the potential for producing adverse emotional outcomes but only in the context of unfulfilled expectations.

Clearly, the extent to which it is possible to generalize from the present study is limited by the size and composition of its sample. However, much of what it reveals is not new and simply confirms the findings of previous work. Principally, there is evidence in the literature both of the heterogeneity of women's perspectives on childbirth and of a strong social class dimension to these orientations. For reasons which Nelson (1983) has explored in some detail, the sociological and feminist literature on childbirth has largely tended to ignore social class differences in women's attitudes towards the experience. In fact, this work has tended to assume that no such differences exist, the implication being that all women share a common perspective on childbirth irrespective of differences in social background. It is also invariably assumed that the model of childbirth to which women subscribe is the 'natural' one. Indeed, some authors have claimed that the medical and natural models of childbirth represent the conflicting views of health professionals and mothers respectively. For example, Graham and Oakley (1981) have argued that, while the medical model predominates among health personnel, most women adhere to a natural perspective on childbirth. They go on to assert that the different and conflicting perspectives of women and health professionals are both a potential and actual source of conflict in maternity settings. Similarly, Nash and Nash have argued that 'In American society at the present time there exist two primary interpretations of the meaning and practice of childbirth: the medical and the 'natural' view' (Nash and Nash, 1979, p. 493).

However, in recent years, the assumption that women share the same natural perspective on childbirth has been seriously challenged. The best example of this is Nelson's work in the United States (Nelson, 1983). She found that the middle- and working-class women in her sample of 322 had very different attitudes towards childbirth. (Social class was distinguished on the basis of differences in levels of educational attainment and not in terms of the traditional classification by occupation.) The middle-class women looked for a pleasurable and rewarding experience, based upon an absence of intervention, and a co-operative – as opposed to instructional – relationship with their medical and midwifery attendants.

The working-class women, on the other hand, placed little value on the experience of childbirth itself. In fact, according to Nelson, they almost never used the word 'experience'. The main focus of their attention was the baby, with labour and delivery being regarded as something merely to be endured. Their approach to the birth was passive, their priority being to get it over with as quickly and painlessly as possible. The middle-class women, in contrast, seldom mentioned pain or length of labour when talking about the birth. Their main concern was to eliminate barriers to a positive experience. The different preferences of the two groups were reflected in their attitudes towards intervention. For example, while 57% of the working-class women indicated a desire for pain relief during labour, only 11% of the middle-class sample did so. Similarly, while 59% of the working-class women expressed a desire for induction through the artificial rupturing of their membranes, the corresponding figure for the middle-class women was only 4%. Nelson describes the contrasting orientations of the two groups of women in the following way:

> The working class women seemed to be striving for speed (enema, episiotomy, artificial rupture of membranes), less pain (medication) and technological safety (delivery room birth, monitoring). They favored intervention because they thought it could bring the product easily, quickly and safely. The middle class women favored a process which entailed safety (as they defined it) and personal participation, but excluded medical intervention in a 'natural' process.... Among middle class women the goal was a childbirth free from the prevailing medical and technological model embodied in the authority of the male physician. Working class women sought freedom from the birth process itself through the use of strategies which would reduce pain and effort. Working class women were not trying to give the experience a unique definition. They were trying to survive it with a minimum of embarrassment, discomfort and isolation (Nelson, 1983, pp. 291–2).

Further evidence of the distinctive perspectives of working-class women is provided by Reid and her colleagues reporting on a British study of childbirth (Reid *et al.*, 1983). They found that, unlike certain middle-class groups, the majority of their working class sample invested little significance in the birth itself and preferred to cede control of the process to medical experts. The women in their study had no desire to have a birth experience: they simply looked forward to having their baby. As Reid and her colleagues put it, 'Many women regarded birth as a physical hurdle to the production of a live baby and not as an act to be enjoyed' (p. 55). Among this group of women there was little opposition to intervention. On the contrary, the fact that the hospital possessed the necessary technology for intervening during labour and delivery was a source of considerable reassurance. Those forms of intervention that eased the process of childbirth for the mother were especially welcome.

The findings of these two studies clearly confirm our own results on working-class views of childbirth. Together with our own, they also demonstrate that there is an important social class dimension to attitudes towards giving birth. Specifically, it would appear that the desire for a natural birth is largely a middle-class phenomenon and that the expectations and priorities of working-class women differ considerably from those of many of their middle-class counterparts. Indeed, the orientations of working-class women would appear to have more in common with the medical model of childbirth than with the natural one. These social class differences may be partly a product of the failure of feminist and natural childbirth literature to reach working-class audiences combined with the fact that the middle-class model of childbirth is largely rooted in movements that are more or less exclusive to that social group (see Nelson, 1983). Certainly, the single, universal model of childbirth promoted in the feminist literature suggests that middle-class feminists are sadly out of touch with the needs and aspirations of working-class women.

I do not, of course, mean to imply by all of this that any particular perspective on childbirth is right or wrong or better or worse than any other. My purpose in this chapter has simply been to document the perspectives of different sections of the population and to thereby increase our knowledge of the ways in which orientations towards childbirth may differ between different social groups. These differences are, of course, not just of academic significance. They also have important implications for the content and organization of maternity services. Three issues stand out as being particularly worthy of attention. First, our respondents' numerous fears about the birth would seem to indicate a need for more antenatal support from midwives and others. In particular, there is a clear need for reassurance and information in relation to pain relief, intervention, parturition and recognition of the onset of labour. Perhaps part of this educative function could be undertaken by community midwives visiting pregnant women at home either as an alternative, or as a supplement, to the information-giving activities in antenatal clinics. Secondly, the study revealed that there is considerable scope for improvement in communication during labour and delivery, particularly in terms of better explanation of the reasons for individual intervention procedures. Above all, though, this chapter has emphasized the need for maternity services to be flexible in their approach and to be as responsive as possible to the varying needs and preferences of all of those whom they serve.

ACKNOWLEDGEMENTS

I would like to record my gratitude to the following colleagues who contributed to the study on which this chapter is based: Andrew Boddy for his help and support throughout; Lynda Wigley and Michelle Myers for assistance in the collection of the data; Rita Dobbs for tireless clerical support; Mary Smalls for computing and statistical assistance; Margaret Reid for earlier comments on the chapter, and Margaret Appleton for excellent secretarial support provided, as always, with such cheerfulness and patience.

I am also most grateful to the staff of Glasgow's maternity hospitals at the Royal Infirmary, the Southern General and Stobhill for granting access to the women and their maternity records. The project would not, of course, have been possible without the willing participation of the 80 mothers who took part and to them we owe a particular debt. Finally, the study was generously supported by a grant from the Scottish Home and Health Department. The Social Paediatric and Obstetric Research Unit is funded by the Scottish Home and Health Department and Greater Glasgow Health Board.

REFERENCES

Arms, S. (1975) *Immaculate deception.* Houghton Mifflin, Boston.

Blehar, M.C. (1979) Preparation for childbirth and parenting. *Families Today, 1,* NIMH Science Monographs 1, 143–70.

Cartwright, A. (1979) *The dignity of labour? A study of childbearing and induction.* Tavistock, London.

Comaroff, J. (1977) Conflicting paradigms of pregnancy: Managing ambiguity in antenatal encounters. In Davis, A. and Horobin, G. (eds), *Medical encounters: The experience of illness and treatment,* Croom Helm, London.

Graham, H. and Oakley, A. (1981) Competing ideologies of reproduction: Medical and maternal perspectives on pregnancy. In Roberts, H. (ed.), *Women, health and reproduction,* Routledge and Kegan Paul, London.

Haire, D. (1978) The cultural warping of childbirth. In Ehrenreich, J. (ed.), *The culture of modern medicine,* Monthly Review Press, New York, pp. 185–201.

Kitzinger, S. (1978) *The experience of childbirth.* Penguin, London.

Lumley, J. (1985) Assessing satisfaction with childbirth. *Birth, 12* (3), 141–5.

Macintyre, S. (1981) *Expectations and experiences of first pregnancy.* Report on a Prospective Interview Study of Married Primigravidae in Aberdeen. Occasional Paper no. 5, Institute of Medical Sociology, University of Aberdeen.

McIntosh, J. (1985) *The birth of the blues: A psycho-social study of postnatal depression.* Report submitted to the Scottish Home and Health Department.

McIntosh, J. (1986) Postnatal blues: A bio-social phenomenon? *Midwifery, 2,* 187–92.

Nash, A. and Nash, J.E. (1979) Conflicting interpretations of childbirth: The medical and natural perspectives. *Urban Life, 7* (4), 493–512.

Nelson, M.K. (1983) Working class women, middle class women and models of childbirth. *Social Problems, 30* (3), 284–97.

Oakley, A. (1975) The trap of medicalised motherhood. *New Society, 34* (689), 639–41.

Oakley, A. (1979) *Becoming a mother.* Martin Robertson, Oxford.

Oakley, A. (1980) *Women confined: Towards a sociology of childbirth.* Martin Robertson, Oxford.

Oakley, A. (1984a) The consumer's role: Adversary or partner? In Zander, L. and Chamberlain, G. (eds), *Pregnancy care for the 1980s,* Royal Society of Medicine, London and Macmillan Press Ltd, London and Basingstoke.

Oakley, A. (1984b) Consumers' revolt. In Oakley, A. (ed.), *The captured womb:*

A history of the medical care of pregnant women, Blackwell, Oxford.

Pitt, B. (1968) Atypical depression following childbirth. *British Journal of Psychiatry, 114*, 1325–35.

Porter, M. and Macintyre, S. (1984) What is, must be best: A research note on conservative or deferential responses to antenatal care provision. *Social Science and Medicine, 19* (11), 1197–1200.

Reid, M.E. (1983) A feminist sociological imagination? Reading Ann Oakley. *Sociology of Health and Illness, 5* (1), 83–94.

Reid, M.E., Gutteridge, S., and MacIlwaine, G. (1983) *A comparison of the delivery of antenatal care between a hospital and a peripheral clinic.* Report submitted to the Scottish Home and Health Department.

Riley, E.D.M. (1977) What do women want? The question of choice in the conduct of labour. In Chard, T. and Richards, M. (eds), *Benefits and Hazards of the New Obstetrics*, Spastics International Medical Publications, Heinemann Medical Books, London.

Topliss, E.P. (1970) Selection procedures for hospital and domiciliary confinement. In McLachlan, G. and Shegog, R. (eds), *In the beginning: Studies of maternity services*, Oxford University Press, Oxford.

CHAPTER ELEVEN

Why don't women breast feed?

Ann M. Thomson

There has been growing concern, particularly in areas of the world where survival rates for babies are poor, at the continuing decline in breast feeding. At its international congress in 1984 the International Confederation of Midwives (ICM) adopted a policy that stated the rights of babies in this respect. These rights are:

The right of all babies to be breast fed for at least the first 6 months of life, especially in parts of the world where malnutrition, morbidity and mortality are prevalent;
The right of all mothers to proper advice, help, encouragement and counselling for successful breast feeding;
The right of all families to accurate information about all aspects of breast feeding (ICM, 1984).

Although a considerable volume of literature exists on factors associated with the incidence of breast feeding, few prospective studies of baby feeding intentions have been undertaken. One such study carried out in the late 1970s (Thomson, 1978) is described in this chapter. The first section of the chapter comprises a review of literature on breast feeding, some of the findings of the study are then presented and considered in the light of subsequent research on this topic.

PREVIOUS RESEARCH ON BREAST FEEDING

Incidence

Concern for the decreasing incidence of breast feeding is not new. In 1720, Dionis in her *Treatise of Midwifery* states that 'if women did their duty as they ought, they would all be Nurses ... but nowadays not only Ladies of Quality, but even Citizens' and ordinary Tradesmen's wives refuse to suckle their children.' Current concern in the United Kingdom (UK) about the declining incidence of breast feeding led to the setting up of a working party to advise on infant feeding policies. The report of this working party (DHSS, 1974) recommended that all mothers be encouraged to breast feed their baby for a minimum of two weeks and preferably for the first four to six months of life. However, several reports have been published that show breast feeding rates very much below the 100% recommended by government. Eastham *et al.* (1976) report a rate of 28%; Bacon and Wylie (1976) 39%; Rice and Seacombe (1975) 52%; and Jones and Belsey (1977) 62%. In Jones and Belsey's (1977) study, the incidence was reduced to 20% by the time the baby was 12 weeks old. Following the publication of their 1974 report, the DHSS requested the Office of Population Censuses and Surveys to undertake a national survey of feeding practices in the first year of life in England and Wales in one month in 1975 (Martin, 1978). This survey showed that 51% of mothers started to breast-feed, at two weeks 35% were breast feeding, but at four months only 13% were breast feeding.

A subsequent survey of feeding patterns in the UK (Martin and Monk, 1982) demonstrated an increase in the incidence of breast feeding in that 65% of women started to breast feed, at two weeks 52% were breast feeding, and at four months 26% were still breast feeding. Martin and Monk (1982) point out that when considering these figures it has to be remembered that the increased number of women starting to breast feed is likely to lead to a higher incidence at subsequent dates. However, they also found that not only did an increased number of women start to breast feed their baby but they continued for longer than did the women in 1978. As encouraging as this information is, it must be remembered that the incidence of 26% breast feeding at four months post-delivery is significantly below that recommended by the DHSS (1974).

Factors associated with the decision to breast feed

A number of authorities accept only a physical reason for not breast feeding, that is the inability to produce and/or deliver an adequate amount of milk to the baby (Shanghai Child Health Centre Coordinating Group, 1975). However, methods of feeding the baby, other than by the breast, is not a new phenomenon, and baby feeding utensils date from the seventeenth century, if not from before (*Nursing Times*, 1976).

Numerous studies, including those by Newson and Newson (1965), Newton and Newton (1967), Grosvenor (1969), Hubert (1974), Bacon and Wylie (1976), Eastham *et al.* (1976), Jones and Belsey (1977), Martin (1978), Hally *et al.* (1981) and Martin and Monk (1982), have been undertaken in an attempt to discover why so many British women do not breast feed. From the results of these studies, it is evident that there are factors other than the inability to produce milk and/or deliver it to the baby that influence a woman against breast feeding. These studies have shown that a high proportion of those who choose to bottle feed their baby come from the lower socio-economic groups, have the minimal amount of educational experience, are younger when having their first baby, are more likely to have been bottle fed themselves, and are unlikely to have a close relative who approves of, or who is encouraging them to breast feed. In the following sections, findings relating to these and other factors are discussed in detail.

Cultural factors. Cultural factors were shown to influence the women in Hubert's (1974) study of pregnancy and childbirth in a working-class London borough. She found that some of the British women had only seen African, West Indian and Gypsy women breast feeding. The respondents considered these groups of women to be their social inferiors so they bottle fed their baby in order not to be associated with them. Conversely, Jones and Belsey (1977) felt that the higher incidence of breast feeding among women in the London borough of Lambeth was possibly due to the example set by the large immigrant population in that area.

Embarrassment. When asked why they are not breast feeding, the most commonly given reason by women was 'embarrassment' (Grosvenor, 1969; Bacon and Wylie, 1976; Eastham *et al*, 1976; and Martin, 1978). Rolls (1973) stated that 'Despite contemporary liberal attitudes towards sex, there is still a widespread notion that breast feeding is embarrassing, indecent and vulgar if it takes place anywhere except in the utmost privacy'. This statement was illustrated by a report in the *New York Times Magazine* (Marlens, 1975) of an event that had occurred in a Miami park. Police had recently arrested three young women after observing them in a socially disruptive activity. The women had been breast feeding. The charge was indecent exposure.

Some women cannot contemplate the idea of breast feeding in front of their husband, mother or women friends (Newson and Newson, 1965) and the baby's older siblings (Eastham *et al.*, 1976). Lack of adequate housing (Grosvenor, 1969) is seen by some to increase this embarrassment because of the impossibility of withdrawing to another room to feed the baby. However, Richards and Bernal (1972) did not find any statistically significant difference in the amount of accommodation available between women who breast fed and those who bottle fed. Richards (1975) has shown, though, that more people were present in the room at a bottle feed than at a breast feed. The bottle feed took on the status of a social event.

Sexual factors. In modern western society, the breast has become a sex symbol. Kinsey *et al.* (1948) stated that there is reason to believe that in our culture, more men are physically aroused by the sight of the naked female breast than by the sight of the naked female genitalia. In everyday life, clothes are generally designed to enhance the female breast, so long as they do not reveal the nipple. However, the nipple is frequently revealed in newspaper and magazine pictures that have captions implying that this is sexually attractive. Although the 'tease' of the partial view of the breast may be acceptable in everyday life, the total exposure of the breast and nipple at breast feeding, which is depicted as being necessary in health education posters and pictures, may be thought to be removing a woman's control of the sexual arousal of men.

There is conflicting evidence on the relationship of breast feeding and sexual intercourse. Newton (1955), when interviewing women during pregnancy, found that those who intended to breast feed desired intercourse less frequently than did those who intended to bottle feed. In their postnatal study Masters and Johnson (1966) found that those who breast fed had a more rapid return to coition than did those who bottle fed. But 25% of the breast feeding women did express guilt feelings because of the admitted sexual stimulation of the sucking process.

The role of women and the advice they are given. Although artificial milks were first produced at the end of the nineteenth century it was not until the 1920s and 1930s that they were widely available. They were hailed as the liberators of women as the mother was no longer required to be tied to her baby. There have been two camps of thought in this respect in the current women's liberation movement. There are those who feel that it is a woman's biological role to breast feed her baby and that she should be given every assistance to make sure that she can (Helsing, 1975); and there are those who feel that the mother should not always have to be the person who feeds and cares for the child (Morgan, 1976). To do this the baby must be, partially at least, bottle fed (Morse and Harrison, 1988); although there have been some personal reports of the advocacy of the return of 'wet nursing'. In her plea not to 'cajole and bully women generally to breast feed', Morgan (1976) describes breast feeding as 'a time-consuming and purposeless charade'. Helsing (1975) suggests that the confusion in a woman's identity, which can affect her decision on how to feed her baby, has been increased by the almost total dominance by men in the field of advice on baby feeding. Fisher (1985) demonstrated that these men were mostly paediatricians who were experts on bottle feeding but their application of the principles of bottle feeding to breast feeding led to the further decline in breast feeding. Helsing (1975) feels that more women might breast feed if women who had themselves breast fed gave the advice to prospective breast feeders.

This view is supported by the research carried out by Ladas (1970). She assessed the effect of support given to breast feeding mothers by the La Leche League in the U.S. The La Leche League is an organization composed of women who have breast fed successfully who give information, support and encouragement to women who are breast feeding for the first time. Ladas (1970) found a significant correlation between the amount of support given and the number of women who started to breast feed, and between a lack of information about breast feeding and the incidence of bottle feeding.

Scoggin (1971) carried out an experiment to assess the effects of an ante- and postnatal educational programme about breast feeding on the incidence of breast feeding. Those in the experimental group attended a class about breast feeding at 36 weeks gestation and were then visited at home at three and ten days postpartum. No contact was made with the women in the control group. When the babies were five months old, 60% of those in the experimental group were breast fed compared with 40% in the control group.

Bacon and Wylie (1976) state that women who bottle feed are less susceptible to advice in general. This, however, should not necessarily be a judgement on the women, as Hubert (1974) has shown that well-intentioned and accurate advice may be given in such a way that less-educated women cannot use it effectively.

Richards and Bernal (1972) showed that women who were unsuccessful with breast feeding were those who had tried to follow the advice that they had been given in hospital. This advice was that the baby should be fed every four hours and that the mother should try to miss out a feed at night. These authors report that those who were successful with breast feeding were those who fed more frequently than the advice had stated. Some women whose baby woke 2–3 hours after a feed interpreted this as a sign of insufficient milk because they were under the impression that a breast feed should satisfy a baby for four hours. Davies and Thomas (1976) in a survey of mothers attending an Infant Welfare Clinic found that the most frequently given reason for early abandonment of breast feeding was 'an insufficient milk supply'. The advice of the professionals to rectify this matter had been to give complementary feeds, and in all cases the milk supply had dried up within two weeks. There appeared to have been no assessment of whether the baby was 'fixed' correctly and was not 'nipple sucking', and no attempt to increase supply by increasing stimulation (Hytten, 1975) or by increasing calorie intake (Whichelow, 1975). It is possible that these women had decided that they wanted to discontinue breast feeding and that this was an excuse that was known to be acceptable to the health professionals in that area. If, however, advice on the correct 'fixing' of the baby at the breast and advice on increasing the milk supply based on the physiology of lactation had been given, it is possible that some women may have been able to continue breast feeding. If the professionals are not giving advice based on scientific principles, the women cannot be blamed for their failure when acting on this advice.

Role models. The size of the 'normal' family in the west has decreased greatly in the last 200 years. In large families older children would see each new baby being breast fed. As the older daughters started their own family, their own mother was just completing hers. Society was much less mobile and it was likely that the daughter would live in close proximity to her mother. These new mothers would have a role model in the form of their own mother to copy when starting to feed their own baby.

Today's new mother is unlikely to have seen breast feeding (Eastham *et al.*, 1976). She is unlikely to be living near her own mother and even if her mother breast fed, Moyes (1976) has shown that her mother is reluctant to give information which she feels is 20 years out of date.

Convenience. In the studies reported by Newson and Newson (1965), Grosvenor (1969), Bacon and Wylie (1976), and Martin (1978), some women gave as their reasons for choosing to breast feed the fact that it was 'more convenient' and 'less trouble' than bottle feeding. But in two of these studies, Grosvenor (1969) and Bacon and Wylie (1976), 'more convenient' and 'less trouble' were also given as reasons for bottle feeding.

Some women feel that breast feeding restricts their social life and that by bottle feeding, someone else is able to feed the baby while they are out for the evening (Grosvenor, 1969; Bacon and Wylie, 1976; Eastham *et al.*, 1976; Martin, 1978). Some women have said that they have bottle fed because their husband wants to feed the baby (Newson and Newson, 1965; Eastham *et al.*, 1976).

Socio-economic status. All studies of the incidences of breast feeding have shown that the women who breast feed come from the higher socio-economic groups (Grosvenor, 1969; Bacon and Wylie, 1976; Eastham *et al.*, 1976; Martin, 1978). The socio-economic group of the mother in these studies was determined by comparing her husband's occupation with the Registrar General's classification. However, Richards and Bernal (1972) feel that to assess the problem on socio-economic status alone could be misleading. They are of the opinion that there is a geographical sub-cultural factor that is involved as well. In their study of mother–child interaction in Cambridge, they found that women who bottle fed their baby had a longer gap between their first and second babies than those who breast fed, in spite of the fact that they were using a less efficient method of contraception. This, they feel, suggests that those who bottle fed either had a lower fertility rate than those who breast fed or they had intercourse less frequently.

Attitudes. Newton and Newton (1950) suggested that attitudes to breast feeding have a relationship to the successful outcome of breast feeding. The respondents in their study were interviewed shortly after birth and independent judges assessed the written records of the interviews and divided the attitudes into three categories. Of those who were considered to have positive attitudes to breast feeding, 74% had enough milk by the fifth day after delivery to make 'formula supplementation' unnecessary, whereas only 35% of those who expressed negative attitudes toward breast feeding had enough milk to make formula supplementation unnecessary at the same time. However, as giving routine formula supplementation interferes with the production of milk by reducing the stimulation of suckling, negative attitudes alone cannot be considered responsible for the unsuccessful breast feeding in this study. Hytten *et al.* (1958) found, in their study of women breast feeding over a period of three months, that there was a higher incidence of breast feeding among those women whose attitudes were not considered to be very positive, but these positive attitudes were not indicative of success. Martin (1978) attempted to assess attitudes to breast and bottle feeding by asking women to consider 26 statements about breast and bottle feeding and to indicate the extent to which they agreed or disagreed with each statement. Following factor analysis, the statements were grouped into three factors: Factor 1 indicated a distaste for breast feeding, Factor 2 indicated that breast feeding is best for babies, and Factor 3 emphasized the convenience of bottle feeding.

Those who started breast feeding had scores for Factors 1 and 2 that were significantly different when compared with the scores of those who started bottle feeding, but the scores for Factor 3 were not significantly different. As this study was carried out six weeks after delivery, the group that had started breast feeding included some women who had already discontinued breast feeding. When the scores for those who had discontinued breast feeding were compared with the group who were still breast feeding at six weeks, the scores for Factor 1 were lower in the group that was still breast feeding than in the group who had discontinued to feed. When Factor 2 was considered, the scores were higher among those who were still breast feeding than among those who had discontinued. Martin (1978) states that it is not possible to assess from this study if the women who stopped breast feeding would have had scores before the baby was born that would have been predictive of their behaviour postnatally, or whether their scores would have changed over time with their behaviour. When the scores for Factor 3 for the group of women who had stopped breast feeding were considered, they differed significantly from those who were still breast feeding but they did not differ significantly from those who did not breast feed at all. Again Martin (1978) suggests that, although it is possible that high scores on this factor may be predictive of stopping breast feeding before six weeks, the results may imply that attitudes to breast feeding of the women who stopped breast feeding changed as a result of their unsuccessful experience. Martin suggests that in an attempt to discover if attitudes to breast feeding before a baby is born are predictive of success or failure, a prospective study should be undertaken.

Other factors. Bacon and Wylie (1976) report that 'return to work and studies' was given by some women as the reason for not breast feeding. Jones and Belsey (1977), however, found that only 11% of women had returned to work within 12 weeks of delivery and several of these were still breast feeding their baby. Martin (1978) also found that the proportion of women who breast fed initially was not significantly related to their working status when the baby was four months old.

Grosvenor (1969), Smith (1969), Richards and Bernal (1972) and Martin (1978) have shown a relationship between the level of education a woman achieved and the breast feeding rate. The higher this level of education, the more likely a woman was to breast feed.

Timing of decision on how the baby was to be fed. Barnes and Barnes (1976), Eastham *et al.* (1976) and Jones and Belsey (1977) have suggested that the decision as to which method of baby feeding will be used is taken early in pregnancy. Of the studies reported here, however, all except one (Richards and Bernal, 1972) investigated the reasons for choice of feeding method after the baby was born, and not at the suggested 'decision time'. Thus, Eastham *et al.* (1976) undertook their research within 48 hours of delivery, Jones and Belsey (1977) carried out their interviews when the baby was 12 weeks old and Barnes and Barnes (1976) postal study was carried out 15–24 months following delivery. It is possible that memory could have adversely affected the recall of events.

As a preliminary to their ethological study of baby feeding, Richards and Bernal recruited the respondents to their study at 38 weeks gestation and investigated reasons for choice of feeding method at this time. In a study of antenatal teaching, Hardie interviewed the respondents at the 20th and 38th week of gestation but she did not enquire about choice of feeding method until the 38th week of gestation (Hardie, personal communication).

If Barnes and Barnes (1976), Eastham *et al.* (1976) and Jones and Belsey (1977) are correct in their assumption that the decision on the method by which the baby will be fed is taken early in pregnancy, then antenatal teaching on this subject, which rarely starts before the 28th week of gestation, is of little value and the DHSS (1974) and Eastham *et al.* (1976) would be correct in recommending teaching about baby feeding in schools to both boys and girls.

In an attempt to assess the need for this teaching the study reported in this chapter comprised an investigation of the following:

1. At what point in relation to pregnancy was the decision taken on how the baby was to be fed?
2. What factors have been shown to influence the decision to breast feed or bottle feed?
3. What were the feeding outcomes?

STUDY DESIGN AND METHODS

As existing studies, which had been undertaken retrospectively, suggested that the decision on how the baby was to be fed was made early in pregnancy, it was necessary to investigate this problem as near the previously suggested decision time as possible. It was felt that the earliest time it would be practicable to recruit a suitable number of women to the study was at the booking visit to the hospital antenatal clinic. Because it is possible that the respondents could have given replies which they thought were expected rather than what they actually intended to do, a longitudinal study following the women up until six weeks post-delivery was designed.

A semi-structured interview schedule was compiled to elicit information in the following areas:

1. demographic details
2. educational experience
3. experience and knowledge of baby feeding
4. where the knowledge of baby feeding was obtained
5. information about and expectations of this pregnancy

In order to assess attitudes to baby feeding, a tool based on the Semantic Differential was designed.

The women were interviewed at the booking clinic, at alternate visits to the clinic during pregnancy, in the postnatal ward, at home three weeks after delivery if the respondent started breast feeding, and all respondents were interviewed at home when the baby was six weeks old. The Semantic Differential tool was administered at recruitment to the study and at six weeks post-delivery (further information on this can be found in Thomson, 1978).

If respondents were recruited during the first trimester of pregnancy and then followed up until six weeks after delivery, there was a possible contact time with the interviewer of 40 weeks. It was felt that this long contact time may have inadvertently supported those who intended to breast feed and have had a 'Hawthorne effect' (Roesthlisberger and Dickson, 1939) on the incidence of breast feeding at six weeks post delivery. In an attempt to control for this, a group of women at any stage of pregnancy was recruited from the routine antenatal clinic and interviewed, in a similar manner, from the time of recruitment until six weeks post-delivery. Although this latter group still had some support during pregnancy, their contact time with the researcher was less.

In order to assess the success or failure of breast feeding at six weeks post-delivery, 'successful' breast feeding was defined as 'breast feeding which was continuing six weeks after the baby's birth, where no regular complementary feeds were being given and where the mother and baby appear satisfied with the outcome of breast feeding'. Occasional supplementary feeds were permitted without affecting the definition 'successful' where these feeds allowed the mother to go out for social occasions or allowed her to have an unbroken night's sleep.

Inclusion criteria

In order to exclude women who had previous experience of feeding their baby, primipara only were recruited to the study. Although it was intended to include single women, it was found during pilot work that women who were not living with the baby's father, or who were not intending to get married were refusing to participate. Therefore only those single women in a stable union or those who said they were intending to get married were included in the study. As the women were to be interviewed at home postnatally, only those living within a ten-mile radius of the centre of the town where the study was undertaken were invited to participate.

Recruitment

All women who attended the booking antenatal clinic during a two-month period who were (i) primiparous; (ii) married, going to get married or living in a stable relationship; and (iii) lived within a ten-mile radius of the centre of the town, were approached and invited to participate. Twenty-nine women fulfilled the criteria; 25 agreed to participate. Hereafter this group is referred to as the 'booking clinic group' (BCG).

To recruit a comparable group at any stage of pregnancy, women were approached at the routine follow-up antenatal clinic. The first woman at the clinic who fulfilled the criteria was invited to participate. If she was willing to participate, and it was convenient for her, she was interviewed straight away, or an appointment was made to interview her at a later date. Following this interview, the next woman at the clinic who came within the criteria was approached. Forty five women fulfilled the criteria; 41 agreed to participate. Hereafter this group is referred to as the 'routine clinic group' (RCG).

The sample

In total, 66 women agreed to take part in this study, 25 in the BCG and 41 in the RCG. In the BCG one woman miscarried early in pregnancy and another delivered a stillborn baby at 36 weeks gestation. Another respondent was in hospital at six weeks post-delivery, but her husband agreed to be interviewed. He said that although his wife had started breast feeding, she had changed to bottle feeding when the baby was five days old.

In the RCG one respondent delivered twins at 27 weeks gestation, one was stillborn and the other lived for two days. Two respondents in this group declined to be interviewed at six weeks post-delivery. Both had been bottle feeding on discharge from hospital, and at the postnatal clinic it was recorded in their medical records that they were bottle feeding.

FINDINGS

The findings from this study are presented in two sections:

1. the timing of the decision about baby feeding made by women in the main study group (the booking clinic group) and factors related to this decision
2. feeding intentions and feeding outcomes of the two groups and factors related to these.

The timing of the decision about baby feeding in the booking clinic group

The 25 women in the BCG were interviewed about baby feeding at their first visit to the hospital antenatal clinic. Twenty-one (84%) of the 25 had decided how they were going to feed their baby, with 18 respondents intending to breast feed and three to bottle feed.

The gestation at which the 21 respondents who had already decided how they were going to feed their baby attended the antenatal clinic for the first time is shown in Table 11.1. Eighteen (72%) were in the first trimester of pregnancy, thus confirming the findings of Barnes and Barnes (1976), Eastham *et al.* (1976) and Jones and Belsey (1977) that women decide how they are going to feed their baby early in pregnancy.

The gestations of the four respondents who had not decided how they were going to feed their baby were 9, 10, 16 and 28 weeks. The reasons they gave for not having made a decision were:

I had a large chest before I got pregnant. I don't know, I would like to breast feed.

I've never thought about it.

I've got too many things on my mind at the moment, I'm getting married in a week.

I don't know why I can't decide, I know breast feeding is better, but I'm not entirely happy.

The two respondents who mention breast feeding and who appear to have heard the pro-breast feeding propaganda both decided to bottle feed. As both had 'shared' antenatal care and did not return to hospital until the 32nd week of gestation, it is not possible to pinpoint exactly the

Table 11.1 Gestation at booking of respondents who knew how they were going to feed their baby

Gestation at booking	Number of respondents
8 weeks	1
9 weeks	4
10 weeks	4
11 weeks	4
12 weeks	1
13 weeks	3
14 weeks	1
15 weeks	1
16 weeks	1
20 weeks	1
Total	21

Source: Compiled by the author.

time at which they made their decision. The respondent who had not thought about baby feeding had a miscarriage. The respondent who could not give any thought to her baby until after her wedding decided to bottle feed before her next visit to the clinic at 33 weeks gestation, her wedding having taken place meantime.

Two of these women who had not decided how they were going to feed their baby when they came to the booking clinic reported discussions with members of the health professions (one a midwife and one a health visitor) who had given them the impression that breast feeding was better than bottle feeding. One respondent had been given the book *You and Your Baby* (published by the British Medical Association) by her GP and had read about baby feeding in there.

Factors that may have affected the timing of a decision about baby feeding

People involved in decision-making

Family and friends. The respondents were asked to state who had discussed baby feeding with them. The replies are shown in Table 11.2 and are grouped according to whether the decision had been made. Some of the respondents had discussed feeding with more than one person. Sixteen (76%) of the 21 who had made a decision had discussed feeding with their husband and 12 had discussed baby feeding with their mother. Three of those who had made a decision had made this decision without discussion with anyone else. All of those who had not made up their mind had discussed the topic with someone – one with her husband, one with her mother, one with her mother and a cousin, and one had discussed baby feeding with friends.

Table 11.2 Whether or not decision was made on feeding by people with whom baby feeding was discussed

Person with whom baby feeding discussed	Decision made (n = 21)		Decision not made (n = 4)
	no.	%	no.
Husband	16	76	1
Mother	12	57	2
Mother-in-law	2	9	0
Friends	8	38	1
Neighbours	4	19	0
Other relatives	5	24	1
None	3	14	0

Source: Compiled by the author.

Health professionals. Of the 25 respondents in the BCG, only three said that a member of the health professions had discussed baby feeding with them before they attended the booking clinic. All three said that their GP had discussed it with them; one also said she had had a discussion with her health visitor. These three women had all made a decision on how they intended to feed their baby. It is not possible to say whether the health professionals played any part in influencing the decision-making of these three women.

Health professionals may influence the public in ways other than by direct contact, for example, by health education in schools, magazine articles, radio and television programmes, and parentcraft books. The respondents were asked if they had attended any parentcraft classes at school; whether they had read anything in books, magazines or news-papers about baby feeding; and whether they had heard anything on the radio or seen anything on the television about baby feeding. Only seven of the respondents could remember the availability of any parentcraft classes at school; six had attended these classes but none could remember any specific teaching on baby feeding. Of the six who had attended these classes, five had made a decision about baby feeding prior to attendance at the booking clinic. Fifteen (60%) of the respondents in the BCG had read something about baby feeding before their first visit to the hospital; two of these respondents had not yet decided how they would feed their baby.

Eleven of those in the BCG had seen programmes on television about baby feeding and all these respondents had made a decision on how they would feed their baby. At the time the respondents were recruited to the study, there was a programme on the television about having a baby.

Witnessing baby feeding and decision-making. Seventeen (68%) of the respondents in the BCG had seen a baby being breast fed, and eight had not. Similar proportions of both groups had decided how they would feed their baby: 82% (14) of the former and 88% (7) of the latter.

Feeding intentions and outcomes for the two groups

Two groups of respondents were investigated in an attempt to discover if the researcher, by interviewing the respondents over a longer period of time, was providing support for those who intended to breast feed. The intentions and practices of the respondents in the two groups are shown in Figs 11.1 and 11.2. The incidences at six days post-delivery have been shown because this was the time that the majority of the respon-dents were discharged from hospital. Incidences of baby feeding at ten days post-delivery have been shown as this was the time at which the midwife handed over the care of the woman to the health visitor.

At six weeks post-delivery, ten of the remaining 23 (43%) respon-dents in the BCG were in fact breast feeding 'successfully', whereas only eight (20%) of the remaining 40 respondents in the RCG were doing so

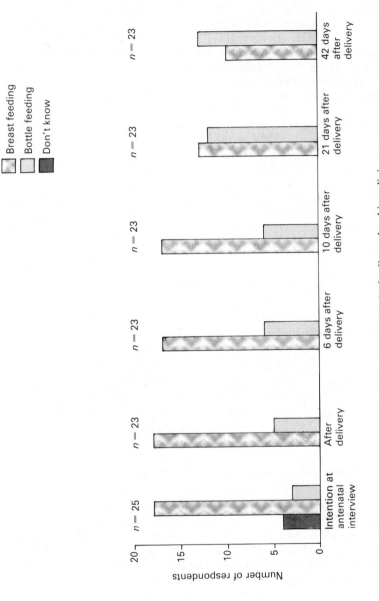

Figure 11.1 Comparison of number of respondents breast or bottle feeding – booking clinic group.

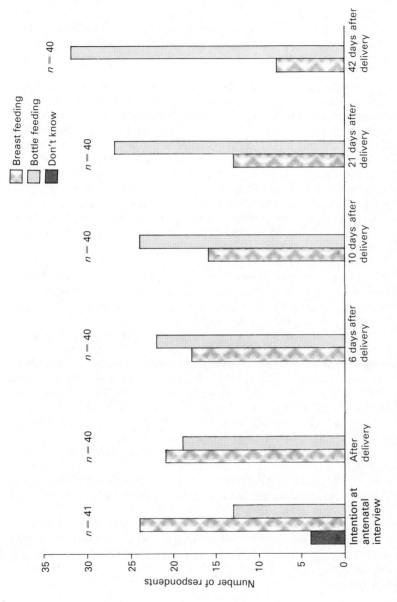

Figure 11.2 Comparison of number of respondents breast or bottle feeding – routine clinic group.

($p < 0.05$). However, although not statistically significant, there had been a higher incidence of intention to breast feed in the BCG (18 (72%) of the respondents) when compared with the RCG, where only 24 (59%) of the 41 respondents had intended to breast feed. Again, although not statistically significant, there was a higher incidence of starting to breast feed in the BCG (78%) when compared with the RCG (55%).

Age, socioeconomic status, level of education and whether the woman had a relative who approved of, or was encouraging her to breast feed appear to have affected the incidence of breast feeding (Newson and Newson, 1965; Newton and Newton, 1967; Grosvenor, 1969; Hubert, 1974; Bacon and Wylie, 1976; Eastham *et al.*, 1976; Jones and Belsey, 1977; Martin, 1978). The two groups in this study were therefore compared on these variables to discover if there was any differences that might account for the differences in incidence of breast feeding. The groups were also compared in terms of how the respondents were fed themselves as a baby, gestation at booking and smoking habits. There were no significant differences between the two groups in any of these respects (Thomson, 1978).

Although there was a higher incidence of breast feeding in the BCG (43%) at six weeks post-delivery when compared with the RCG (20%), this outcome cannot be attributed solely to the support/influence of the increased contact with the researcher, as there was a higher incidence of 'intention to breast feed' in the BCG.

Taking the two groups together, the incidence of breast feeding steadily declined and consequently the converse is true of bottle feeding. Thus at the initial recruitment interview, 42 (64%) of the 66 respondents intended to breast feed their baby, 16 (24%) intended to bottle feed, and 8 (12%) had not yet decided how they would feed. Of the 63 respondents who delivered a live baby, 39 (62%) started to breast feed after delivery and 24 (38%) started to bottle feed. At six weeks post-delivery, only 18 (29%) respondents were breast feeding 'successfully'.

Although the prevalence of breast feeding at six weeks post-delivery is slightly higher than the 24% found by Martin (1978), it is about the same as the 32% found by Martin and Monk (1982) in Scotland, where this study was undertaken, and is considerably below the level recommended by government (DHSS, 1974).

As the two groups were so similar in terms of the range of characteristics described and in terms of feeding intentions and outcomes, data from the two groups in relation to factors affecting the decision of how a baby will be fed and factors affecting method of feeding are presented together.

Factors affecting the decision of how a baby will be fed

At the first interview, all respondents in this study were asked how they intended to feed their baby. Forty-two of the women intended to breast feed, 16 to bottle feed, and eight had not decided how they would feed their baby.

Reasons for choosing to breast or bottle feed. Table 11.3 shows the respondents' reasons for choosing to breast feed and the percentage giving each reason. All those intending to breast feed gave at least one reason for their choice, and some gave several.

Table 11.4 shows the reasons the respondents gave for choosing to bottle feed. Apart from 'convenience', they are all reasons for not breast feeding, not positive reasons for bottle feeding. Three of those intending to bottle feed 'did not know' why they had made their choice, while some of the others gave several reasons.

The most frequently given reasons for intending to breast feed were that 'breast milk is better/safer for the baby', and that 'breast feeding is the natural way to feed a baby'. 'Embarrassment' at the thought of feeding in front of other people and in particular 'other men' was the most frequently given reason for bottle feeding.

Influence of family and friends on the decision. The number of people who had talked with the respondents, grouped according to feeding intention, is shown in Table 11.5. Nine of the women had not discussed baby feeding with anyone and all said they had decided how they would feed their baby; four were going to breast feed, five to bottle feed. Forty-nine of the 66 women (74%) had discussed baby feeding with their husband. The next person with whom breast feeding was most frequently discussed was the respondent's own mother (55%).

Table 11.3 Reasons given by the respondents for intending to breast feed

Reason	Number (n = 42)	
	no.	*%*
Breast milk is better/safer for the baby (protects against illness, less risk of cot death, etc.)	32	76
It's the natural way to feed	16	38
Closer or different relationship with the baby	11	26
It's more convenient (easier or quicker)	8	19
Cheaper	4	10
Always wanted to breast feed	3	7
Less risk of infection from dirty feeding utensils	2	5
Other (instinct, disapproval of relatives, persuasion by TV, etc.)	6	14

Source: Compiled by the author.

Table 11.4 Reasons given by the respondents for intending to bottle feed / not to breast feed

Reason	Number (n = 16) no.	%
Embarrassment	12	75
Convenience (especially when going out)	4	25
'Just don't want to do it'	4	25
When breast feeding, only the mother can feed the baby	2	12
Awareness of 'personal tension' and possible effect on let-down reflex	2	12
Concern over amount of milk that the baby gets	3	19
Put off by other people's bad experiences	2	12
Other	5	31
Don't know	3	19

Source: Compiled by the author.

Table 11.5 Intended feeding method by people with whom feeding method discussed

People with whom baby feeding discussed	Intended feeding method				
	Breast (n = 42) no.	Bottle (n = 16) no.	Don't know (n = 8) no.	Total (n = 66) no.	%
Your husband	35	9	5	49	74
Your mother	21	9	6	36	55
Your husband's mother	11	5	1	17	26
Friend(s)	16	8	3	27	41
Neighbour(s)	5	4	–	9	14
Other mothers at the clinic	5	3	–	8	12
Other relatives	11	3	2	16	24
None	4	5	–	9	14

Source: Compiled by the author.

Those who intended to breast feed were more likely than those who intended to bottle feed to have discussed feeding with their husband (83% compared with 56%), but the proportions were similar with regard to discussing feeding with their mother.

How the respondents were fed as babies. Previous research has shown that women who bottle fed their baby were more likely to have been bottle fed themselves than breast fed. Fifty one (77%) of these women knew how they had been fed (Table 11.6). There is a statistically significant relationship between knowledge of how the respondent was fed and the choice of baby feeding method; women intending to breast feed were more likely to have been breast fed themselves than women who were intending to bottle feed ($p < 0.01$), and women who were intending to bottle feed were more likely to have been bottle fed themselves than those who were intending to breast feed ($p < 0.01$).

Although there was a tendency for those who intended to breast feed to be older, have a higher level of education, and to be less likely to smoke, these findings were not statistically significant.

Factors affecting method of feeding at six weeks post-delivery

The women's reasons for abandoning breast feeding are shown in Table 11.7. Eleven of the women gave up because they said they had an inadequate milk supply. However, the diagnosis of lack of supply has to be questioned as there appeared to be a lack of understanding on the part of the women, and the midwives advising them, on the physiology of lactation. Some of the respondents had asked their advisors if they could feed for longer periods but were told, 'no, because a baby gets what it wants in 20 minutes sucking and after that he just wants to play'. Others did not think it was right to feed more frequently than every four hours because that was what they had been taught in the hospital.

Some women stated they had received conflicting advice. This appeared in particular to come from community midwives and is illustrated by the following quote:

> when we were given the fourth set of advice from the fourth person in four days we [mother and baby] were both totally confused.

Table 11.6 Intended feeding method by how fed as a baby

Feeding method as a baby	Intended feeding method							
	Breast		Bottle		Don't know		Total	
	no.	%	no.	%	no.	%	no.	%
Breast	27	79	5	38	–	–	32	63
Bottle	7	21	8	62	4	100	19	37
Total	34	100	13	100	4	100	51	100

Source: Compiled by the author.

Table 11.7 Respondents' reasons for abandoning breast feeding

Reasons	Respondents who abandoned breast feeding	
	no.	%
Problems with nipples	3	14
Too much milk	2	9
Too little milk	11	52
Problems with baby not sucking	3	14
Abscess	1	5
Mother to go into hospital for surgery	1	5
Total	21	100

Source: Compiled by the author.

In an attempt to elicit factors related to this decline in breast feeding, comparison of some factors known to affect a respondent's choice of feeding method was made between those respondents who were 'success-ful' with breast feeding, those who were 'unsuccessful', and those who bottle fed. At the end of the study 18 (29%) of the remaining 63 respondents were breast feeding 'successfully', 21 (33%) had started to breast feed but had changed to bottle feeding and were therefore cat-egorized as 'unsuccessful' breast feeders, and 24 (38%) had started to bottle feed.

Although there was a tendency for those who were breast feeding 'successfully' to be older than those who were 'unsuccessful', this differ-ence was not statistically significant. When the social class of the woman's partner was considered, there was a much higher incidence of 'successful' breast feeding among those women whose husband had a non-manual occupation when compared with those who were 'unsuccessful' with breast feeding ($p < 0.05$) and those who bottle fed ($p < 0.05$) (Table 11.8) (Two women were unable to give sufficient information about their husband's job for social class to be assigned.) The 'successful' breast feeders also had a higher level of education as judged by 'age on leaving school' (Table 11.9) and attendance at further education (Table 11.10).

In an attempt to discover if events surrounding labour and delivery had any relationship to the incidence of breast feeding, type of labour (spontaneous, accelerated or induced), length of labour, type of delivery and analgesia during labour were examined in relationship to feeding method at six weeks post-delivery. None was found to be related.

Table 11.8 Feeding method at six weeks post-delivery by social class

Social class	Method of feeding					
	'Successful' breast feeding		*'Unsuccessful' breast feeding*		*Bottle feeding*	
	no.	*%*	*no.*	*%*	*no.*	*%*
Non-manual (1–3M)	12	67	6	30	7	30
Manual (3M–5)	6	33	14	70	16	70
Total	18	100	20	100	23	100

Source: Compiled by the author.
N.B. Two women were unable to give sufficient information about their husband's occupation for their social class to be determined.

Table 11.9 Feeding method at six weeks post-delivery by age on leaving school

Age on leaving school	Method of feeding					
	'Successful' breast feeding		*'Unsuccessful' breast feeding*		*Bottle feeding*	
	no.	*%*	*no.*	*%*	*no.*	*%*
14 years	–	–	–	–	1	4
15 years	5	28	8	38	9	38
16 years	3	17	10	48	12	50
17 years	4	22	2	10	2	8
18 years	6	33	1	5	–	–
Total	18	100	21	100	24	100

Source: Compiled by the author.

Research has shown that those who breast feed their baby within one hour of delivery have a higher incidence of breast feeding when the baby is one month old (Salariya *et al.*, 1978). In this study only one woman suckled her baby while she was still on the delivery bed. For the remaining 38 women, the time of the first breast feed varied between 1 and 48 hours after delivery but the time of the first feed did not have any relationship with the incidence of 'successful' feeding in this group of women. Attendance at Mothercraft classes did not have any relationship with the type of feeding at six weeks post-delivery.

Table 11.10 Feeding method at six weeks post-delivery by attendance at courses of 'further education'

Attendance at further education	Method of feeding					
	'Successful' breast feeding		'Unsuccessful' breast feeding		Bottle feeding	
	no.	%	no.	%	no.	%
Yes	16	89	14	67	10	42
No	2	11	7	33	14	58
Total	18	100	21	100	24	100

Source: Compiled by the author.

CONCLUSIONS AND IMPLICATIONS OF DATA

This study was undertaken during a Scottish Home and Health Department Research Training Fellowship. There were constraints, as with all research, on the time and money that were available for this study. As it was considered important to try to identify the time, in relationship to childbirth, when women make the decision about how they will feed their baby, it was important to begin the study as near the decision time, as identified by existing authors, as was feasible. In order to counteract the possibility of the respondents giving information that they thought was required, instead of what they actually intended to do (as demonstrated by Newson and Newson, 1965), a prospective study was designed so that actual feeding practices could be examined. This meant that the length of the study for each woman could be up to 40 weeks if she booked for antenatal care as early as eight weeks gestation. Consequently, the number of women who could be studied was small. This has obvious implications for the interpretations that can be placed on the findings. At the time this study was undertaken, there was no existing study of baby feeding practices that had attempted to examine the subject as near the suggested time the decision on baby feeding method was made. Two large studies of baby feeding have been published subsequently (Martin and Monk, 1982; Hally *et al.*, 1981), but only one (Hally *et al.*, 1981) examined the subject during pregnancy and did not start until the 34th week of gestation.

This study has confirmed the suggestions of previous authors (Barnes and Barnes, 1976; Bacon and Wylie, 1976; Eastham *et al.*, 1976; Martin, 1978) that the decision on how a baby will be fed is made early in pregnancy, if not before conception. Of the 21 women in the BCG who had made a decision at the time of their first visit to the hospital antenatal clinic about how their baby would be fed, 18 (72%) were in the first trimester of pregnancy. Very few of the respondents had had direct contact with health professionals, but indirect contact by means of books, magazines, newspapers or the television had been made. The DHSS (1974) and Eastham *et al.* (1976) are therefore correct in suggesting that teaching on the best method to feed a baby is too late when given in pregnancy and should be undertaken at the only other time when prospective parents are a captive audience – at school. As this study and others (Eastham *et al.*, 1976; Martin, 1978; Hally *et al.*, 1981) have demonstrated that the prospective father has an influence on the baby feeding method adopted, then the classes in school should be for boys as well as girls.

As in other studies (Bacon and Wylie, 1976; Eastham *et al.*, 1976; Martin, 1978; McIntosh, 1985), the reasons given for breast feeding were that it was better for the baby and the natural way to feed. The major reason for bottle feeding was that breast feeding would be embarrassing. There was a feeling among the respondents in this study who intended to bottle feed that they would not want to breast feed in front of other people. As in Richards and Bernal's study (1972) there was no difference in the amount of accommodation available to the women in the groups of intended feeding method at recruitment to the study. However, Grosvenor (1969) and two subsequent studies (Hally *et al.*, 1981; McIntosh, 1985) found that accommodation that does not allow women privacy appears to be encouraging women not to breast feed. Richards (1975) found that there were more people present at a bottle feed than at a breast feed.

The proportion of women breast feeding fell dramatically in this study from 64% intending to breast feed at the time of recruitment to the study, to 29% breast feeding successfully at six weeks post-delivery. This is considerably less than that recommended by the DHSS (1974). A subsequent study has shown no change in the six week incidence of breast feeding at 25% (Hally *et al.*, 1981). In a national study, Martin and Monk (1982) found an incidence of breast feeding of 42% in England and Wales in 1980, but for Scotland, where this study was undertaken, it was 32%. McIntosh, in a study of a small sample of women in the lower socioeconomic groups in Glasgow, found the incidence of breast feeding at six weeks post-delivery to be 34%. It would therefore appear that the incidence of breast feeding is not rising in Scotland as in other parts of the United Kingdom.

Other authors (Graham and McKee, 1980; Oakley, 1980, 1981) have commented that the reasons for abandoning breast feeding are multi-factorial. The major reason women gave for abandoning breast feeding in this study and in others (Newson and Newson, 1965; Eastham *et al.*, 1976; Martin and Monk, 1982; McIntosh, 1985) was an insufficient milk supply. But Houston (1984) has stated, 'It is unlikely that such large numbers of women are in fact incapable of producing enough milk for their babies.'

Short (1976) suggests that genetic selection would have eliminated those women physiologically incapable of producing milk. The women in this study were subjected to a hospital breast feeding policy that took no account of the physiology of lactation. They were only allowed to feed every four hours and only for restricted times at each feed. They were also required to give a complementary feed after each breast feed. They were therefore not giving adequate stimulation to the breast to produce enough milk to meet the baby's needs. The routine giving of complementary feeds for the first three days can only have confused the baby's sucking pattern, diminished his appetite and further reduced his stimulation of the breast to produce milk. These women were therefore programmed to fail, and those who managed to succeed, despite the odds, were to be congratulated. There has been an increase in midwifery literature recently about factors that enhance the incidence of breast feeding. One of these factors is the so-called 'demand' feeding, in which the baby is fed when the baby is hungry and not when the clock says he is. However, Martin and Monk (1982) and McIntosh (1985) have shown that rigid feeding regimes are still in existence in some maternity hospitals.

Although the incidence was very much less than the incidence of 'insufficient milk', the second most common reason for abandoning breast feeding was 'sore nipples'. Illingworth and Stone (1952) showed that a rigid feeding regime, such as the one in use where this research was undertaken, contributed to the incidence of sore nipples. It did not decrease the incidence, as its protagonists claim. Woolridge (1986a,b) has shown the importance of 'fixing' the baby correctly to the breast at each feed. If the mother is not told the importance of this, then soreness, perhaps even cracks will ensue. It is pointless trying to encourage more women to breast feed until midwives can correctly assist those women who already start to breast feed satisfactorily.

Two-thirds of the women who stopped breast feeding in this study did so after the midwife had ceased her daily visits. Houston (1984) demonstrated the value of postnatal support, whether it be from friends and family, lay support groups or health professionals, to the breast feeding woman. It would therefore seem sensible for health professionals to assess a woman's support system postnatally and, if it appears inadequate, to provide one for as long as it is necessary. It is pointless for health professionals in general and midwives in particular to state that 'breast is best' and then not provide the necessary 'advice, help, encouragement and counselling' (ICM, 1984). That, as Clark (1976) suggests, is providing 'lip service only'.

REFERENCES

Bacon, C.J. and Wylie, J.M. (1976) Mothers' attitudes to infant feeding at Newcastle General Hospital in summer 1975. *British Medical Journal, 1,* 308–9.

Barnes, D. and Barnes, P. (1976) Infant feeding 1. *Nursing Times, 72* (31), 1210–1211.

Clark, J. (1976) Lip service only. *Nursing Mirror, 140* (3), 39–40.

Davies, D.P. and Thomas, C. (1976) Why do women stop breast feeding? *Lancet, 1,* 420.

Department of Health and Social Security (1974) *Present day practice in infant feeding.* HMSO, London.

Dionis (1720) *A general treatise of midwifery,* London.

Eastham, E., Smith, D., Poole, D. and Neligan, G. (1976) Further decline of breast feeding. *British Medical Journal, 1,* 305–7.

Fisher, M.C. (1985) How did we go wrong with breast feeding? *Midwifery, 1* (1), 48–51.

Graham, H. and McKee, L. (1980) *The first months of motherhood.* Health Education Monograph Series no. 3, London.

Grosvenor, P. (1969) Influences affecting mothers' decisions about infant feeding. Unpublished MSc thesis, University of Edinburgh.

Hally, M. (1981) *A study of infant feeding: Factors influencing choice of method.* Health Care Research Unit, University of Newcastle upon Tyne.

Helsing, E. (1975) Women's liberation and breast feeding. *Journal of Tropical Paediatrics and Environmental Child Health, 21* (5), 290–2.

Houston, M. (1984) Home support for the breast feeding mother. In Houston, M. (ed.), *Maternal and infant health care,* Churchill Livingstone, Edinburgh.

Hubert, J. (1974) Belief and reality – social factors in pregnancy and childbirth. In Richards, M.P.M. (ed.), *The integration of a child into a social world,* Cambridge University Press, Cambridge.

Hytten, F.E. (1975) The physiology of lactation. Paper presented at DHSS symposium, published by Newman, London.

Hytten, F.E., Vorsten, J.C. and Thomson, A.M. (1958) Difficulties associated with breast feeding. *British Medical Journal, 1,* 310.

Illingworth, R.S. and Stone, D.G.H. (1952) Self-demand feeding in a maternity unit. *Lancet, i,* 682.

International Confederation of Midwives (1984) *Policy on baby feeding.* ICM, London.

Jones, R.A.K. and Belsey, E.M. (1977) Breast feeding in an inner London borough – a study of cultural factors. *Social Science and Medicine, 11,* 175–9.

Kinsey, A.C., Pomeroy, W.B. and Martin, C.E. (1948) *Sexual behaviour in the human male.* W.B. Saunders, Philadelphia.

Ladas, A.K. (1970) How to help mothers breast feed. *Clinical Paediatrics, 9* (12), 702–5.

McIntosh, J. (1985) Barriers to breast feeding: Choice of feeding method in a sample of working class primiparae. *Midwifery, 1* (4), 213–24.

Marlens, A. (1975) Macho about pocketbooks. *New York Times Magazine,* July 27.

Martin, J. (1978) *Infant feeding 1975: Attitudes and practice in England and Wales.* OPCS, London.

Martin, J. and Monk, J. (1982) *Infant feeding 1980.* OPCS, London.

Masters, W.H. and Johnson, V.E. (1966) *Human sexual response.* Little Brown, Boston.

Morgan, P. (1976) Breast feeding – the mystic maternal cult. *New Society, 36,* 413–4.

Morse, J.M. and Harrison, M.J. (1988) Patterns of mixed feeding. *Midwifery, 4* (1), 19–23.

Moyes, B. (1976) Perceptions of pregnancy. Unpublished PhD thesis, University of Edinburgh.

Muller, M. (1974) *The baby killer.* War on Want, London.

News Feature (1976) Pap boats and bubby pots. *Nursing Times, 72* (45), 1748–9.

Newson, J. and Newson, E. (1965) *Patterns of infant care in an urban community.* Pelican, London.

Newton, N. (1955) *Maternal emotions: A study of women's feelings towards menstruation, pregnancy, childbirth, breast feeding, infant care and other aspects of femininity.* Hoeber, New York.

Newton, N. and Newton, M. (1950) Relationship of ability to breastfeed and maternal attitudes toward breast feeding. *Paediatrics, 5,* 869–75.

Newton, N. and Newton, M. (1967) Psychological aspects of lactation. *New England Journal of Medicine, 277,* 1179–88.

Oakley, A. (1980) *Women confined. Towards a sociology of childbirth.* Martin Robertson, Oxford.

Oakley, A. (1981) *From here to maternity.* Penguin, Harmondsworth.

Rice, R.H. and Seacome, M. (1975) Attitudes of a group of mothers to breast feeding, Part 1. *Midwife, Health Visitor and Community Nurse, 11,* 175–9.

Richards, M.P.M. (1975) Feeding and the early growth of the mother–infant interaction. In Kretchner, N. *et al.* (eds), *Milk and lactation — Modern problems paediatric,* Karger, Basel.

Richards, M.P.M. and Bernal J.F. (1972) An observational study of mother–infant interaction. In Blurton-Jones, N. (ed.), *Ethological studies in child behaviour,* Cambridge University Press, Cambridge.

Roethlisberger, F.J. and Dickson, W.L. (1939) *Management and the worker.* Harvard University Press, Harvard.

Rolls, R. (1973) Breast feeding (letter). *British Medical Journal, 4* (5890), 493.

Salariya, E.M., Easton, P.M. and Cater, J.I. (1978) Duration of breast-feeding after early initiation and frequent feeding. *Lancet, ii,* 1141–3.

Scoggin, J.P. (1971) The effects of learning on breast feeding success. Unpublished Master's thesis, Arizona State University.

Shanghai Child Health Care Coordinating Group (1975) Measurement of growth and development of infants under 20 months in Shanghai. *Journal of Tropical Paediatrics and Environmental Child Health, 21* (5), 284–9.

Short, R.V. (1976) Lactation. The central control of reproduction. In CIBA Foundation Symposium 45, *Breast feeding and the mother,* Elsevier, Amsterdam.

Smith, D.V. (1969) Attitudes to breast feeding (letter). *British Medical Journal, 2* (5685), 695.

Thomson, A.M. (1978) Why don't women breast feed? Unpublished report to Scottish Home and Health Department, Edinburgh.

Whichelow, M. (1975) Calorie requirements for successful breast feeding. *Archives of Diseases of Childhood, 50,* 669.

Woolridge, M. (1986a) The 'anatomy' of infant sucking. *Midwifery, 2* (4), 164–171.

Woolridge, M. (1986b) Aetiology of sore nipples. *Midwifery, 2* (4), 172–5.

Index